Keto Desserts:

100+ Ketogenic Diet Dessert Recipes You'll Die For!

Kevin Gise © 2018

Disclaimer:

This book is for informational purposes only and the author, his agents, heirs, and assignees do not accept any responsibilities for any liabilities, actual or alleged, resulting from the use of this information.

This report is not "professional advice." The author encourages the reader to seek advice from a professional where any reasonably prudent person would do so. While every reasonable attempt has been made to verify the information contained in this eBook, the author and his affiliates cannot assume any responsibility for errors, inaccuracies or omissions, including omissions in transmission or reproduction.

Any references to people, events, organizations, or business entities are for educational and illustrative purposes only, and no intent to falsely characterize, recommend, disparage, or injure is intended or should be so construed. Any results stated or implied are consistent with general results, but this means results can and will vary. The author, his agents, and assigns, make no promises or guarantees, stated or implied. Individual results will vary and this work is supplied strictly on an "at your own risk" basis.

Introduction

Thanks for purchasing my book "Keto Desserts: 100+ Ketogenic Diet Dessert Recipes You'll Die For!"

I hope you like keto dessert recipes I've included. There are so many wonderful dessert recipes to try out on the keto diet. These quick and easy recipes should have you covered.

Let's begin!

Almond & Chocolate Fat Bombs (Serves 12)

Ingredients:

1/2 cup of Unrefined Coconut Oil

1/2 teaspoon of Vanilla

3 tablespoons of Heavy Whipping Cream

1/2 cup of Almond Butter

2 tablespoons of Truvia

3 tablespoons of Cocoa Powder

Pinch of Salt

Directions:

1. In your small-sized saucepan, add your nut butter and coconut oil. On a low heat, melt these together.

2. Add your cocoa powder, heaving whipping cream, truvia, and vanilla.

3. Take off the heat and put into a pouring container.

4. Line your cupcake tin with cupcake liners, or use a silicone mold. Pour out in 12 equal portions.

5. Place into your freezer for about 15 minutes to harden.

6. Store in your refrigerator or freezer in a tightly sealed container.

Nutrition Facts:

Carbs: 2 grams

Calories: 156

Almond, Coconut, & Coconut Fat Bombs

Ingredients:

1 stick of Butter + 2 tablespoons of Butter

8 ounces of Raw Coconut Butter

8 ounces of Unsweetened Almond Butter

1 bar of 85% Cocoa Chocolate

Sweetener

Optional Add-Ins

Roasted Nuts

Cocoa Nibs

Unsweetened Coconut Flakes

Dried Unsweetened Fruit

Directions:

1. In your microwave-safe bowl, soften your stick of butter, the coconut butter and the almond butter for 1 to 3 minutes until they are easy to stir together. Once your butters are blended, add in any extra add-ins making sure there is still enough butter blend to coat everything. Add sweetener if desired. Stir together well.

2. The butter mix then needs to be put in your silicone molds. Make a ganache by melting your chocolate bar in your microwave in a glass dish. Add your 2 tablespoons of butter to make it smooth and creamy.

3. Dip your chilled fat bombs in the chocolate and allow it to cool on a piece of wax paper or a silicone sheet. Drizzle the melted chocolate over each fat bomb. Store in your refrigerator.

Baked Apples (Serves 4)

<u>Ingredients:</u>

2 ounces of Butter (Room Temperature)

1 Tart or Sour Apple

1-ounce of Pecans

1/2 teaspoon of Ground Cinnamon

4 tablespoons of Coconut Flour

1/4 teaspoon of Vanilla Extract

<u>Directions:</u>

1. Preheat your oven to 350 degrees.

2. Mix your soft butter, chopped nuts, coconut flour, cinnamon, and vanilla into a crumbly dough.

3. Rinse your apple, but don't peel it or remove the seeds. Cut off both ends and cut the middle part in four slices.

4. Place your slices in a greased baking dish and add dough crumbs on top. Bake for approximately 15 minutes or more or until the crumbs turn golden brown.

5. Add heavy whipping cream and vanilla to a medium-sized bowl and whip until soft peaks form.

6. Allow the apples to cool for a couple of minutes and serve with a dollop of whipped cream.

Nutrition Facts:

Calories: 345

Net Carbs: 7 grams

Fat: 33 grams

Blackberry Mascarpone Bombs (Serves 9)

Ingredients:

1/2 teaspoon of Lemon Juice

1/2 cup of Blackberries

1/2 teaspoon of Liquid Stevia

2 tablespoons of Mascarpone Cheese

1 cup of Coconut Butter

1/4 teaspoon of Vanilla Extract

1 cup of Coconut Oil

Directions:

1. Start by thawing your blackberries in a small-sized bowl.

2. Once your blackberries are thawed place your mascarpone cheese, lemon juice, coconut oil, coconut butter, vanilla extract, and liquid stevia in your mixing bowl and mix on low until everything is combined well.

3. Spoon into your silicone cupcake liners.

4. Freeze for approximately 30 minutes and keep refrigerated.

Nutrition Facts:

Net Carbs: 4 grams

Calories: 437

Butter Pecan Ice Cream (Serves 6)

<u>Ingredients:</u>

2 Egg Yolks

2/3 cups of Chopped Pecans

1 cup of Heavy Cream

1/3 cup of Erythritol

1 teaspoon of Vanilla Extract

1 pinch of Stevia

2 tablespoons of Butter

1/8 teaspoon of Xanthan Gum

<u>Directions:</u>

1. Melt your butter in your pan over a low flame. Allow to brown slightly.

2. Add in your cream and allow it to simmer.

3. Turn your heat to the lowest setting, adding your erythritol. Allow to completely dissolve. Stir gently.

4. Transfer your mixture into a large-sized mixing bowl. Add Stevia. Use your electric hand mixer to get your ingredients combined.

5. While mixing on the medium setting, add your xanthan gum to allow your ingredients to thicken and bind.

6. In another small-sized bowl, separate your egg yolks and add in your vanilla extract. Slowly beat them into your mixing bowl as you're beating the cream mixture.

7. Add your chopped pecans and fold in using a spoon.

8. Place your bowl in your freezer. Take out to stir every 40 minutes so pecans are well incorporated.

9. Allow to freeze for at least 3 hours before serving.

Nutrition Facts:

Protein: 2 grams

Fat: 20 grams

Carbs: 1 gram

Calories: 200

Cake Batter Cookies (Serves 12)

Ingredients:

Cookies:

1/4 cup of Softened Butter

1 Egg

1/2 teaspoon of Xanthan Gum

1 cup of Sukrin Gold

1/4 cup of Erythritol

1 Egg Yolk

1 1/2 teaspoons of Butter Extract

1 teaspoon of Vanilla Extract

1/4 teaspoon of Almond Extract

2 tablespoons of Rainbow Sprinkles

1/2 teaspoon of Salt

3/4 cup of Almond Flour

1 tablespoon of Coconut Flour

Optional Filling:

1/4 cup of Softened butter

1/2 cup of Sukrin Melis

Directions:

1. Cream together your erythritol, Sukrin Gold, and softened butter with electric hand mixer.

2. Mix in your egg yolk and egg.

3. Add butter, almond, and vanilla extracts.

4. Add your salt and flours. Mix it well until it is combined.

5. Add your xanthan gum. Mix until your batter thickens.

6. Mix in your sprinkles and stir to evenly distribute them.

7. Refrigerate batter for an hour.

8. Lay out your saran wrap and place the cookie batter onto it.

9. Wrap your batter into log 3-inches thick. Make sure the thickness is uniform throughout. Refrigerate 2 hours to allow to harden.

10. Take out of your refrigerator and preheat your oven to 350 degrees. Unwrap your log and roll to get rid of flattened edges. Slice log into desired cookie thickness. For this example, I cut them into 12 cookies.

11. Line your cookies on a baking sheet lined with parchment paper and cook for approximately 10 minutes. Cookies are done when slightly golden.

12. Allow your cookies to cool down.

13. You can make the optional filling above combining two ingredients. Then put on top of a cookie and place another cookie on top making into a cookie sandwich.

Nutrition Facts:

Calories: 175

Protein: 3 grams

Fat: 17 grams

Carbs: 2 grams

Caramel Chocolate Cake (Serves 4)

Ingredients:

1/4 cup of Carolyn's Low-Carb Caramel Sauce

1/8 teaspoon of Powdered Stevia

1 teaspoon of Vanilla Extract

1/4 cup of Erythritol

4 Medium Eggs

1/2 teaspoon of Cinnamon

1/4 teaspoon of Salt

1/4 cup of Melted Butter

1/2 cup of Cocoa Powder

<u>**Directions:**</u>

1. Prepare your caramel sauce and allow it to cool. Put some in your small-sized jar and allow it to freeze.

2. Preheat your oven to 350 degrees.

3. Prepare your lava cake batter. Combine all of your dry ingredients and mix together to get out any lumps.

4. Combine your wet ingredients and mix with your dry ingredients.

5. Spray 4 ramekins with oil or use butter to grease them.

6. Fill your ramekins halfway each with your batter.

7. Place a tablespoon of caramel sauce into center of each of your ramekins, allowing it to rest on your lava cake batter.

8. Pour the rest of your batter over the caramel. Cover it completely.

9. Place your ramekins on a baking sheet and bake for approximately 13 minutes. Tops of your cake should be set but still jiggle.

10. Allow to relax for approximately 3 minutes. Run a sharp knife around the edges of the ramekin to loosen your cakes.

11. Place your plate upside down onto your ramekin. Flip your ramekin and plate so your ramekin is now facing upside down on your plate. Tap the ramekin to make your cake gently fall onto your plate.

12. Add your desired optional toppings.

Nutrition Facts:

Calories: 230

Protein: 8 grams

Carbs: 6 grams

Fat: 24 grams

Cheesecake Blueberry Popsicles

Ingredients:

2 cups of Cool Whip 95% Fat-Free Whipped Topping

2 cups of Fresh Blueberries

1/2 cup of Light Cream Cheese

6 tablespoons of Icing Sugar

Directions:

1. Puree your blueberries, cream cheese, and icing sugar in your blender until smooth.

2. Gently fold in your whipped topping.

3. Spoon into your popsicle molds and freeze until firm.

4. Run your mold under hot water to loosen popsicles so they are easy to remove.

Chia Chocolate Pudding (Serves 2)

Ingredients:

1 cup of Unsweetened Almond Milk or Skim Milk

3 tablespoons of Chia Seeds

1/4 cup of Fresh or Frozen Raspberries

1 scoop of Chocolate Protein Powder or Cocoa Powder

1 teaspoon of Honey (Only if not using the Protein Powder)

Directions:

1. Mix your chocolate protein powder and almond milk together. Make sure you've stirred it well.

2. Add in your chia seeds. Make sure you've stirred it in well.

3. Let your mix rest for approximately 5 minutes and then stir.

4. Stir again approximately 5 minutes later.

5. Let mix rest for approximately 30 minutes in your refrigerator.

6. Add your raspberries on the top.

<u>Nutrition Facts:</u>

Calories: 235

Protein: 30 grams

Carbs: 19 grams

Fat: 12 grams

Chocolate Cherry Cheesecake

Ingredients:

2 ounces of Heavy Cream

1 tablespoon of Dutch Process Cocoa Powder

8 ounces of Softened Cream Cheese

1 tablespoon of Da Vince Sugar-Free Cherry Flavored Syrup

3 to 5 drops of EZ-Sweet Liquid

1 teaspoon of Stevia Glycerite

Directions:

1. Mix all your ingredients together except for the EZ-Sweet and then whip it into a pudding-like consistency.

2. Add your EZ-Sweet a drop one at a time to your mixture until it is sweet. Spoon your mixture into small-sized serving cups and refrigerate until it sets.

Chocolate Chip & Almond Butter Fat Bombs (Serves 20)

Ingredients:

1/3 cup of Golden Monk Fruit Sweetener

3/4 cup of Almond Butter (Room Temperature)

1/2 cup of Chocolate Chips

1/2 cup + 2 tablespoons of Coconut Oil (Room Temperature)

1 teaspoon of Pure Vanilla Extract

1 1/4 cup of Almond Flour

Directions:

1. Line your 8×8 baking pan with parchment or wax paper.

2. To your medium-sized microwave-safe bowl, add your almond butter and microwave until soft, approximately 15 to 20 seconds.

3. To your bowl of softened almond butter, add your almond flour, coconut oil, monk fruit sweetener, and vanilla extract. Using an electric mixer, mix all your ingredients together until well-combined. (If your almond butter or coconut oil is not incorporating well, place your bowl in the microwave for approximately 10 to 15 seconds to soften your mixture.)

4. To mixture, gently fold in your chocolate chips until they are fully incorporated.

5. To prepared baking pan, pour in your mixture and spread using your spatula until the mixture sits in an even layer.

6. Transfer the pan to your refrigerator and refrigerate for 2 hours.

7. Remove from your refrigerator, cut your bars into the desired size.

Nutrition Facts:

Net Carbs: 2.1 grams

Calories: 193

Chocolate Chip Cheesecake

<u>Ingredients:</u>

8 ounces of Softened Cream Cheese

2 ounces of Heavy Cream

1 teaspoon of Stevia Glycerite

1 teaspoon of Splenda

1 ounce of Mini Chocolate Chips

<u>Directions:</u>

1. Mix all your ingredients together and then whip it into a pudding-like consistency.

2. Spoon your mixture into your small-sized serving cups and refrigerate until it sets.

Chocolate Chip Peanut Butter Ice Cream

Ingredients:

3 Large Egg Yolks

3/4 cup of Sugar-Free Chocolate Chips

1/2 cup of Almond Milk

1/4 cup of Erythritol

1 teaspoon of Vanilla Extract

1/2 cup of Peanut Butter

1/2 cup of Heavy Cream

1/4 teaspoon of Xanthan Gum

1 tablespoon of Vodka (Optional)

Directions:

1. Heat your erythritol and heavy cream on a stove over a low heat. Don't boil. Let it come to a gentle simmer.

2. While that's heating up, whisk together your egg yolks and add in your vanilla extract.

3. Temper the eggs so they don't scramble by slowly adding hot cream while continuing to whisk.

4. Pour the tempered eggs into your hot cream and whisk over a low flame.

5. Add in your xanthan gum and mix until everything thickens up.

6. Transfer to your bowl and add the vodka if you're using it. Chill until it is cooled down.

7. Once your mixture is cool, add to your ice cream maker and follow the instructions for that machine.

8. Once your ice cream is thick in your ice cream maker, add your chocolate chips. In last few seconds of churning, add in your peanut butter.

9. Place in your freezer for a firmer consistency.

Nutrition Facts:

Calories: 295

Protein: 8 grams

Fat: 26 grams

Carbs: 6 gram

Chocolate Coconut Candies (Serves 20)

<u>Ingredients:</u>

<u>Chocolate Topping:</u>

1 ounce of Unsweetened Chocolate

1 1/2 ounces of Cocoa Butter

1/4 cup of Cocoa Powder

1/4 teaspoon of Vanilla Extract

1/4 cup of Powdered Swerve Sweetener

<u>Coconut Candies:</u>

1/2 cup of Coconut Butter

3 tablespoons of Powdered Swerve Sweetener

1/2 cup of Coconut Oil

1/2 cup of Unsweetened Shredded Coconut

Directions:

1. For the candies, line your mini-muffin pan with 20 mini paper liners.

2. Combine your coconut butter and coconut oil in a small-sized saucepan over a low heat. Stir until melted and smooth and then stir in your shredded coconut and sweetener until combined.

3. Divide your mixture among prepared mini muffin cups and freeze until firm, approximately 30 minutes.

4. For the chocolate coating, combine your cocoa butter and unsweetened chocolate together in a bowl set over a pan of simmering water (do not let the bottom of the bowl touch the water). Stir until melted.

5. Stir in your sifted powdered sweetener, then stir in your cocoa powder, until smooth.

6. Remove from your heat and stir in your vanilla extract.

7. Spoon your chocolate topping over a chilled coconut candies and allow it to set, approximately 15 minutes.

8. Candies can be stored on your counter for up to a week.

Nutrition Facts:

Net Carbs: 1 gram

Calories: 240

Chocolate Covered Maple Pecan Bacon (Serves 13)

Ingredients:

Bacon Base:

13 slices of Bacon

1 tablespoon of Maple Extract

2 tablespoons of Erythritol

Coating:

1/4 cup of Chopped Roasted Pecans

4 tablespoons of Unsweetened Cocoa Powder

15 drops of Liquid Stevia

2 tablespoons of Erythritol

Directions:

1. Preheat your oven to 400 degrees. Lay your 13 slices of bacon onto a baking sheet lined with foil.

2. Sprinkle 1 tablespoon of erythritol and 1 1/2 teaspoon of maple extract over one side of the bacon and rub it in.

3. Flip your bacon onto the other side and do the same thing. Rub everything in well.

4. Bake your bacon for approximately 40 to 50 minutes until crisp.

5. Once your bacon is finished, set to the side for 5 minutes to allow it to cool for a moment.

6. In a container, render your bacon fat by tipping cooking sheet at an angle. This should get you about 5 tablespoons of bacon fat.

7. Add 4 tablespoons of cocoa powder, 2 tablespoons of erythritol, and 15 drops of liquid stevia to the bacon grease and mix together well.

8. Transfer your chocolate mixture to a different container so that you can dip the bacon inside. Submerge all the bacon into your chocolate and transfer to a sheet of parchment paper. Sprinkle 1/4 cup of chopped pecans over the bacon before chocolate dries.

9. Put the chocolate covered bacon into your refrigerator for at least 5 hours.

<u>Nutrition Facts:</u>

Calories: 75

Net Carbs: 0.75 grams

Chocolate Covered Strawberries

Ingredients:

1/2 pound of Fresh Strawberries

2 ounces of Chocolate Chips

1 tablespoon of Coconut Oil

2 tablespoons of Coconut Butter

Directions:

1. Melt your chocolate chips. Stir well.

2. Remove from any heat and add in your coconut oil and coconut butter until everything is melted. Move to a small-sized bowl.

3. Dry your strawberries. Grab by stem and dip into the chocolate.

4. Place your chocolate strawberries on a baking sheet lined with parchment paper and refrigerate for approximately 1 hour.

Chocolate Strawberry Mousse (Serves 1)

Ingredients:

1/3 cup of Heavy Whipping Cream

1 Strawberry

4 Drops of EZ-Sweet

1/2 Scoop of Chocolate Whey Powder

2.5 grams of Unsweetened Cocoa

Flakes of 90% Chocolate

Directions:

1, Measure your cream into a container.

2. Add your EZ-Sweet.

3. Add your strawberry.

4. Add your powder.

5. Add your chocolate flakes.

6. Mix 1 to 2 minutes till stiff.

<u>Nutrition Facts:</u>

330 Calories

Protein: 10 grams

Fat: 33 grams

Carbs: 12 grams

Cinnamon Butter Fat Bombs

Ingredients:

1 tablespoon of Cinnamon

1 pound of Grass-Fed Salted Butter

1 1/2 teaspoons of Vanilla Extract

1/4 cup of Honey

Directions:

1. Allow your butter to soften.

2. Add your butter, cinnamon, honey, and vanilla extract to your food processor. Process for a couple of minutes to mix your ingredients and achieve a slightly whipped taste. Stop your food processor as necessary to scrape down the bowl and reincorporate ingredients.

3. Spoon your butter mixture into silicone molds. Alternatively, you can line a cutting board or flat surface with your parchment paper and then spoon dollops of your butter mixture onto your parchment paper.

4. Freeze for an hour or two, then remove from your parchment paper or molds and store in a container in your freezer.

Cinnamon Coconut Peanut Butter Cookies (Serves 15)

<u>Ingredients:</u>

1 cup of Peanut Butter

1 Egg

1/2 teaspoon of Vanilla Extract

1/4 cup of Butter

1/2 cup of Erythritol

2 tablespoons of Shredded Coconut

1 tablespoon of Cinnamon

Pinch of Salt

Directions:

1. Preheat your oven to 350 degrees. Beat together your butter, peanut butter, erythritol, and egg.

2. Add your cinnamon, shredded coconut, salt and fold it all in together.

3. Roll into balls about 1 1/2 inches in diameter. Lay out on a baking sheet lined with parchment paper.

4. Sprinkle with your shredded coconut.

5. Bake approximately for 15 minutes. Edges should become golden colored.

6. Allow it to cool.

Nutrition Facts:

Calories: 140

Protein: 4 grams

Fat: 12 grams

Carbs: 2 grams

Clean Almond Butter Fat Bombs (Serves 12)

Ingredients:

1/4 cup of Almond Flour

2 tablespoons of Mesquite Meal

1 cup of Almond Butter

1 tablespoon of Melted Unrefined Virgin Coconut Oil

1/2 teaspoon of Vanilla Extract

1/4 cup of Coconut Flakes

4 Dates

Directions:

1. Combine all of your ingredients in your food processor.

2. Roll out 1-ounce balls and place them on your parchment-lined baking sheet. Note: If your almond butter has a runny consistency, throw your combined ingredients in the refrigerator or freezer before rolling them into individual balls.

3. Roll your balls into the topping of your choice.

4. Store in your refrigerator or freezer.

Coconut Blackberry Fat Bombs (Serves 16)

Ingredients:

1 cup of Coconut Butter

1 tablespoon of Lemon Juice

1/4 teaspoon of Vanilla Powder or 1/2 teaspoon of Vanilla Extract

1 cup of Coconut Oil

1/2 teaspoon of Sweet Leaf Stevia Drops

1/2 cup of Fresh or Frozen Blackberries

Directions:

1. Place your coconut butter, coconut oil, and blackberries (if frozen) in a pot and heat over a medium heat until well combined.

2. In your food processor or small blender, add your coconut oil mix and remaining ingredients. Process until smooth. Separation may occur if coconut oil mixture is too hot. If using fresh berries, there is no need to cook them with the coconut oil and butter.

3. Spread out into a small-sized pan lined with parchment paper (I used a 6x6-inch container)

4. Refrigerate for one hour or until your mix has hardened.

5. Remove from your container and cut into squares.

6. Store covered in your refrigerator.

Nutrition Facts:

Carbs: 3 grams

Fat: 19 grams

Calories: 170

Coconut Macaroons (Serves 10)

Ingredients:

4 Egg Whites

4 1/2 teaspoons of Water

1 teaspoon of Vanilla

2 cups of Unsweetened Coconut

1/2 teaspoon of EZ-Sweet

Directions:

1. Combine your egg whites and liquids.

2. Add your coconut and mix together.

3. Spread on your greased pie pan.

4. Preheat your oven to 375 degrees. When you put in your macaroons reduce heat to 325 degrees and bake for approximately 14 minutes.

<u>Nutrition Facts:</u>

Calories: 88

Protein: 2 grams

Fat: 8 grams

Carbs: 3 grams

Coconut Raspberry Slice (Serves 20)

Ingredients:

Biscuit Layer:

1 Large Egg

2 cups of Almond Meal

1 tablespoon of Butter (Room Temperature)

1/2 teaspoon of Baking Soda

Coconut Layer:

1 cup of Unsweetened Coconut Milk (Canned)

1/3 cup of Powdered Erythritol

1/4 cup of Coconut Oil

1 teaspoon of Vanilla Bean Powder

3 cups of Unsweetened Desiccated Coconut

Pinch of Sea Salt

<u>Raspberry Layer:</u>

1 cup of Raspberries

3 tablespoons of Chia Seeds

1 teaspoon of Powdered Erythritol

2 tablespoons of Water

<u>Chocolate Layer:</u>

4 ounces of 85% Dark Chocolate

Directions:

1. Preheat your oven to 350 degrees. Combine all your biscuit layer ingredients in a bowl and mix until your dough forms.

2. Line an 8×8 inch baking dish or brownie pan with your parchment paper. Evenly press your biscuit dough into the dish to form the base. Bake in the oven for approximately 15 minutes, until lightly browned and cooked through. Allow it to cool.

3. Make your raspberry layer by adding all of your ingredients into a small-sized pan and stir over a low heat. Break up your raspberries as they cook so a jam forms. Keep stirring for around 5 minutes, until thickened. Allow it to cool.

4. On a medium heat mix your coconut milk and coconut oil until combined.

5. Mix all of your remaining ingredients for the coconut layer together. Add your coconut milk and oil mixture to the dry ingredients and combine well.

6. Add your coconut mixture to your cooled biscuit base and spread evenly. Place in your freezer until set (around 1 hour). Once the coconut layer is hard, spread the raspberry layer over the top of it and return to the freezer to set (around 1 hour).

7. Break your chocolate bar into small-sized pieces, then place in a suitable bowl and melt in your microwave (approximately 3 minutes). Pour your chocolate onto the raspberry layer and return to the freezer to set.

8. Remove from your freezer around 30 minutes before serving. The slices can be stored in the refrigerator for around a week or in the freezer for around 3 months.

<u>Nutrition Facts:</u>

Calories: 240

Net Carbs: 3.5 grams

Protein: 4.5 grams

Coconut Strawberry-Filled Fat Bombs (Serves 15)

Ingredients:

1/3 cup of Coconut Butter

1/3 cup of Diced Fresh Strawberries

1 tablespoons of Unsweetened Shredded Coconut

1/2 tablespoon of Cocoa Powder

1/3 cup of Coconut Oil + 1 tablespoon

8 to 10 drops of Liquid Stevia

Directions:

1. In your bain-marie, add your coconut butter, 1/3 cup of coconut oil, cocoa powder, and a few drops of liquid stevia. Heat until fully melted.

2. Meanwhile, in your small-sized frying pan, add your fresh strawberries and a few spoonfuls of water. Cook over a medium heat until soft. Mash with a fork. Add the berries to a blender with 1 tablespoon of melted coconut oil and a few more drops of liquid stevia. Blend until smooth.

3. Fill your molds with the melted coconut mixture. Add about 1 teaspoon of the strawberry mixture into each mold. Sprinkle with a few shreds of unsweetened coconut.

4. Place in your refrigerator until fully hardened; at least a couple of hours or overnight. Pop out of the molds and store in an air-tight container in the refrigerator.

Nutrition Facts:

Net Carbs: 1 gram

Calories: 106

Coconut White Chocolate Fudge (Serves 24)

Ingredients:

4 ounces of Cacao Butter

1 teaspoon of Coconut Liquid Stevia

1/2 cup of Vanilla Protein Powder

1/2 cup of Coconut Oil

1 cup of Coconut Butter

15-ounce can of Coconut Milk

1 teaspoon of Vanilla Extract

Pinch of Salt

Optional:

Unsweetened Coconut Flake

Directions:

1. Melt your cacao butter in your saucepan over a low heat.

2. Stir in your coconut milk, coconut oil, and coconut butter.

3. Continue to stir until completely smooth, no lumps.

4. Turn off your heat and whisk in protein powder, vanilla extract, stevia, and salt.

5. Pour your mixture into a parchment lined 8x8 pan.

6. Sprinkle with coconut flakes if desired.

7. Refrigerate for 4 hours or overnight.

8. Does not need to be kept refrigerated for storage.

Nutrition Facts:

Net Carbs: 1.2 grams

Calories: 175

Coffee Cake Cinnamon Collagen Fat Bombs (Serves 12)

Ingredients:

1/4 cup of Almond Butter

1/2 cup of Coconut Oil

1 tablespoon of Instant Coffee

1 packet of Vanilla Collagen

1 teaspoon of Cinnamon

Directions:

1. In your small-sized saucepan heat coconut oil and almond butter on low until melted.

2. Microwave your coconut oil for approximately 30 seconds until melted.

3. Stir together all of your ingredients.

4. Pour into an 8x8 pan, mini muffin tins, or silicone/plastic candy molds. Freeze until firm.

Cream Cheese Clouds (Serves 24)

Ingredients:

8 ounces of Softened Cream Cheese

1/2 teaspoon of Vanilla

1/2 cup of Softened Unsalted Butter

3/4 cup of Granular Splenda

Directions:

1. Beat everything with your electric mixer until fluffy.

2. Drop bite-size spoonfuls onto your wax paper-lined baking sheet.

3. Freeze until firm, at least 1 hour. Store in your freezer and eat frozen.

Nutrition Facts:

Net Carb: 1 gram

Calories: 70

Fat: 7 grams

Cream Cheese Peanut Butter Fat Bombs

Ingredients:

3/4 cup of Softened Peanut Butter

4 ounces of Softened Cream Cheese

2 tablespoons of Softened Butter

1 tablespoon of Lemon Juice

3/4 cup of Almond Flour

1/4 cup of Swerve Icing

Directions:

1. Line 12 mini muffin tins with your paper liners and set to the side. You can also use your ice cube tray.

2. In your medium-sized bowl, combine your softened cream cheese, butter, and peanut butter until completely smooth. Add your almond flour, lemon juice, and sweetener and whisk until combined. Evenly distribute into the prepared muffin tins.

3. Place in your freezer for at least 1 hour. Once frozen, transfer the fat bombs to a Ziploc bag for better storing. Keep them in the freezer for up to 3 months.

Crisp Meringue Cookies (Serves 18)

Ingredients:

4 Large Egg Whites

1/2 teaspoon of Almond Extract

1/4 teaspoon of Cream of Tartar

6 tablespoons of Swerve Confectioners

Pinch of Salt

Directions:

1. Preheat your oven to 210 degrees. Pour your egg whites into your mixing bowl, then add your cream of tartar.

2. Start your mixer slowly and increase towards a medium speed. When your egg whites start to look frothy stop the mixer and add 3 tablespoons of Swerve, the almond extract, and salt.

3. Mix on a high speed until your egg whites whip up to a medium consistency. Stop your mixer and add the remaining 3 tablespoons of Swerve.

4. Continue to whip on a high speed until your meringue becomes very stiff and starts to pull away from the sides of the bowl. Stop the mixer and scrape the meringue out of the whisk and down the sides of the bowl, then mix it again to make sure that everything is mixed evenly.

5. Load your meringue into a piping bag fitted with a large star-shaped tip. Depending on the size of your bag you may need to refill the bag a few times in order to work your way through the entire batch.

6. Place sheets of parchment paper on 2 to 3 baking sheets. How many you need will depend on how closely you can comfortably pipe the cookies next to each other. Pipe out 18 rosette shapes, or whatever shape you prefer.

7. Bake your meringue cookies for approximately 40 minutes at 210 degrees. Once they are done turn the oven off and crack the door open, then allow them to cool for another 30 minutes.

<u>Nutrition Facts:</u>

Calories: 4

Net Carbs: 0.09 grams

Double Chocolate Bundt Cake (Serves 8)

<u>Ingredients:</u>

<u>White Chocolate Glaze:</u>

2 tablespoons of Heavy Cream

3 tablespoons of Powdered Erythritol

1 teaspoon of Vanilla Extract

2 ounces of Anthony's Organic Cocoa Butter Wafers

<u>Bundt Cake:</u>

3 Large Eggs

2 cups of Anthony's Almond Flour

1 cup of Butter

1 1/2 teaspoons of Baking Soda

2 tablespoons of Coconut Flour

1/2 cup of Sour Cream

1 cup of Erythritol

1 cup of Water

1/2 teaspoon of Salt

2 teaspoons of Vanilla Extract

1/2 cup of Cocoa Powder

Topping:

20 grams of Anthony's Organic Cocoa Nibs

Directions:

1. Preheat your oven to 350 degrees.

2. Whisk together 2 cups of Anthony's Blanched Almond Flour with your baking soda, salt, coconut flour, and erythritol.

3. Heat up your butter, water, and cocoa powder in a small pot over medium heat. Whisk until it is combined and then take off heat.

4. Pour half your chocolate mixture into your dry mix and stir it to combine. Once it thickens, pour in other half and stir to combine again.

5. Add 1 egg at a time to your mixture.

6. Add your vanilla extract and sour cream. Stir well.

7. Pour your mixture into a greased bundt cake pan. Bake approximately 40 to 50 minutes.

8. Prepare glaze while cake bakes. Melt your cocoa butter wafers.

9. Add powdered erythritol and stir to combine. Add heavy cream and place in refrigerator. Take out and stir approximately every 5 minutes.

10. Once opaque and thick, blend in blender until it is smooth.

11. Once your cake is done baking, allow it to cool in its pan for approximately 10 minutes. Invert onto a cooling rack on your baking sheet or plate. Allow it to completely cool.

12. Glaze your cake. While your glaze is wet, sprinkle your cocoa nibs over your cake. Allow the glaze to cool down and harden.

Nutrition Facts:

Calories: 520

Protein: 10 grams

Fat: 50 grams

Carbs: 5 grams

Fat Bomb Popsicles (Serves 6)

Ingredients:

1 cup of Organic Blueberries

1 tablespoon of Lakanto Sugar Substitute

1 tablespoon of Vanilla Extract

1/2 cup of Organic Raspberries

3 cups of Coconut Cream (Divided)

Directions:

1. Get 6 popsicle molds and fill the bottom with some of the blueberries, dividing them evenly amongst the 6.

2. In your food processor, blend 2 cups of room temperature coconut cream with the vanilla and the Lakanto. Process until smooth, then pour into your molds, just enough to cover the blueberries by about 1/4 inch. Set the rest to the side at room temperature so it does not separate. If it starts separating, just warm up briefly and blend again.

3. Stick your popsicle sticks in to the molds and place the molds in the freezer until your mixture is almost solid, about 1 hour.

4. Mix your remaining cup of coconut cream and the raspberries in the food processor to create a smooth cream.

5. Pour about 1/2 inch of red mixture in the molds and freeze again for an hour.

6. Next pour another layer of white cream and freeze.

7. Continue with alternate red and white stripes until the top of the mold.

8. Freeze until solid, for at least 3 hours.

9. When ready to eat take out of the freezer and run some hot water over the molds for approximately 20 to 45 seconds, until you are able to free the popsicle.

Nutrition Facts:

Net Carbs: 5.3 grams

Calories: 379

Fudge Macadamia Chocolate Fat Bombs (Serves 6)

<u>Ingredients:</u>

2 ounces of Cocoa Butter

2 tablespoons of Unsweetened Cocoa Powder

2 tablespoons of Swerve

4 ounces of Chopped Macadamias

1/4 cup of Heavy Cream or Coconut Oil

<u>Directions:</u>

1. Melt your cocoa butter in your small-sized saucepan in a bath of water.

2. Add your cocoa powder to your saucepan.

3. Add your Swerve and mix well until all your ingredients are well blended and melted.

4. Add your macadamias and stir it together well.

5. Add your cream, mix well and bring back to temperature.

6. Pour in your molds or paper candy cups.

7. Allow it to cool, then put in your refrigerator to harden.

8. Keep at room temperature, with a slightly softer consistency than chocolate.

Nutrition Facts:

Carbs: 3 grams

Calories: 265

Fudge Mint Fat Bombs

Ingredients:

1 1/5 cups of Nut or Seed Butter

2 tablespoons of Vanilla

1/2 cup of Dried Parsley Flakes

1 1/2 cups of Coconut Oil

1/4 tablespoon of Salt

1 teaspoon of Peppermint Extract

1/2 cup of Sweetener

Melted Chocolate

Directions:

1. Melt your coconut oil in a small-sized saucepan. Add your remaining ingredients to your blender, add your coconut oil and blend until smooth.

2. Pour into an 8x8 baking pan and freeze until solid.

3. Store in your refrigerator to prevent softening.

Ginger Lime Coconut Fudges

<u>Ingredients:</u>

1/2 cup of Condensed Milk

2 1/2 cups of White Chocolate Chips

1/2 cup of Shredded Coconut

1/2 teaspoon of Salt

Zest of 1 Lime (Grated)

Knob of Fresh Ginger (Grated)

<u>Directions:</u>

1. Dry-toast your shredded coconut in a skillet over a medium fire until golden and fragrant, approximately 2 minutes. Set to the side.

2. Combine your chocolate chips and condensed milk in a medium-sized bowl and heat in your microwave for 90 seconds. Stir to combine and heat another 15 seconds. Stir and heat an additional 15 seconds, only if necessary. There should be a few pieces of unmelted white chocolate in your bowl.

3. Stir with a wooden spoon until almost smooth. Add your grated zest, ginger, and toasted coconut and stir well to combine. Scoop onto a parchment lined tray. Spread with a spatula to approximately 1-inch thickness, you can sprinkle the top with additional coconut. Refrigerate until ready to serve. Slice into 1-inch rectangles and store in an airtight container in the refrigerator for up to one week.

Gingerbread Creme Brulee (Serves 6)

Ingredients:

1 3/4 cups of Heavy Whipping Cream

4 Egg Yolks

2 teaspoons of Pumpkin Pie Spice

1/4 teaspoon of Vanilla Extract

2 tablespoons of Erythritol

1/2 Clementine (Optional)

Directions:

1. Preheat your oven to 360 degrees.

2. Separate your eggs by cracking them and placing whites and yolks in separate bowls. Discard the yolks.

3. Add your cream to a saucepan and bring to a boil along with the spices, vanilla extract, and sweetener.

4. Add the warm cream mixture into your egg yolks, a little at a time, while whisking.

5. Pour into oven-proof ramekins or small Pyrex bowls nestled in a larger baking dish with sides. Add water to your larger dish until it's about halfway up the ramekins. The water makes the cream cook gently and evenly for a creamy and smooth result.

6. Bake in your oven for about 30 minutes. Remove your ramekins from the baking dish and allow it to cool.

7. Add clementine on top.

<u>Nutrition Facts:</u>

Calories: 274

Net Carbs: 3 grams

Gluten Free Banana Bread (Serves 8)

<u>Ingredients:</u>

<u>*Dry Ingredients:*</u>

3/4 teaspoon of Cinnamon

1 teaspoon of Baking Powder

1/2 teaspoon of Salt

1/8 teaspoon of Cayenne

1/2 teaspoon of Baking Soda

1 1/3 cup of Almond Flour

1 teaspoon of Xanthan Gum

<u>*Wet Ingredients:*</u>

3 Ripe Bananas

1 Juiced Orange

2 tablespoons of Coconut Oil

1/4 cup of Honey

1/4 teaspoon of Vanilla Extract

Pinch of Orange Zest

Fold-Ins:

3/4 cups of Flax Seeds

3/4 cup of Chopped Walnuts

1/4 teaspoon of Grated Fresh Ginger

2 Grated Carrots

Topping:

Honey

Coconut Butter

Directions:

1. Preheat your oven to 410 degrees.

2. Mash your bananas until a thick wet mush.

3. Add orange zest and juiced orange.

4. Add in vanilla extract, honey, and coconut oil.

5. Add in all your dry ingredients.

6. Shred your ginger and carrots. Fold into mixture. Roughly chop walnuts. Throw into your mixture.

7. Fold in the rest of ingredients.

8. Grease your medium-sized bread pan with some butter or coconut oil. Pour in your batter. Feel free to sprinkle on sugar or drizzle some honey at the end.

9. Bake for approximately 25 minutes at 410 degrees. Lower temperature to 350 degrees and bake for approximately 30 minutes.

10. Allow it to cool and then slice bread.

<u>Nutrition Facts:</u>

357 Calories

Protein: 8 grams

Fat: 24 grams

Carbs: 23 grams

Grasshopper No-Bake Bars

Ingredients:

Mint Layer:

4 cups of Organic Shredded Unsweetened Coconut

2 Hass Avocados

3/4 cup of Melted Coconut Oil

1/4 teaspoon of Salt

1/2 cup of Sweetener

3/8 teaspoon of Organic Peppermint Extract

6 scoops of Stevia

3/4 teaspoon of Vanilla

Chocolate Layer:

1/2 cup of Coconut Oil

1/2 teaspoon of Vanilla

1/2 cup of Cocoa Powder

1/8 teaspoon of Salt

1/4 cup of Xylitol

<u>Directions:</u>

<u>Mint Layer:</u>

1. Lightly grease your 8x8 pan.

2. Place all of your ingredients in high powered blender or a food processor. Process until blended. If you prefer the texture of coconut in the finished result, do not process completely.

3. Spread your mixture into your prepared pan and place in your freezer.

<u>Chocolate Layer:</u>

1. In your small-sized saucepan, melt your coconut oil and sweetener over a low heat.

2. Remove from your heat, add in the remaining ingredients, and stir to combine.

3. Pour over your chilled bottom layer. Return to your freezer until the chocolate layer is solid.

4. Cut into bars.

5. Store covered in the refrigerator or freezer.

Homemade Chocolate Chips (Serves 3)

Ingredients:

1 Low-Carb Chocolate Bar

Directions:

1. Melt your chocolate bar.

2 Pour chocolate onto silicone pot holder.

3. Place in freezer and allow to freeze approximately 2 hours.

4. When frozen, twist your silicone molds and pop out your chips onto a plate.

Nutrition Facts:

Calories: 28

Protein: 0.2 grams

Fat: 2.8 grams

Carbs: 0.1

Homemade Nutella (Serves 12)

Ingredients:

2 cups of Hazelnuts

1/4 cup of Cocoa Powder

1 tablespoon of Coconut Oil

1/2 cup of Erythritol

1/4 cup of Heavy Cream

1/4 cup of Water

1 teaspoon of Vanilla Extract

1/4 teaspoon of Salt

Directions:

1. Preheat your oven to 325 degrees.

2. Spread your cookie sheet and spread hazelnuts evenly on one layer. Roast approximately 10 to 15 minutes.

3. Allow your nuts to cool. Put your nuts in a towel and rub them vigorously.

4. Once nuts have skins off, drop them into your food processor. Blend for a few minutes until it looks like peanut butter.

5. If sticking to sides add a little coconut oil and scrape down the sides.

6. Add in the rest of your ingredients. Continue to blend and scrape the sides.

7. Remove from blender once thoroughly mixed and place in a container.

Nutrition Facts:

Calories: 162

Protein: 3 grams

Ice Cream Fat Bomb (Serves 5)

<u>Ingredients:</u>

4 yolks from Pastured Eggs

4 Whole Pastured Eggs

1/3 cup of Melted Coconut Oil

1/3 cup of Melted Cacao Butter

2 teaspoons of Vanilla Bean Powder

1/3 cup of Xylitol or 15 to 20 drops of Alcohol-Free Stevia

1/4 cup of MCT Oil

8 to 10 Ice Cubes

<u>Directions:</u>

1. Add all your ingredients but the ice cubes into the jug of your high powered blender. Blend on high for approximately 2 minutes, until creamy.

2. While your blender is still running, remove the top portion of the lid and drop in 1 ice cube at a time, allowing your blender to run about 10 seconds between each ice cube. The goal here is to dilute the mixture just a bit and make it cold so it will run through the ice cream maker easier.

3. Once all of your ice has been added, pour the cold mixture into your ice cream maker and churn on high for approximately 20 to 30 minutes, depending on your ice cream maker. If you do not have an ice cream maker, transfer the mixture to your 9x5 loaf pan and place in your freezer. Set your timer for approximately 30 minutes before taking it out to stir. Repeat for 2 to 3 hours, until desired consistency is met.

4. Serve immediately as soft-serve or scoop into a 9x5 loaf pan and freeze for approximately 45 minutes. Store covered in your freezer for up to a week.

Instant Pot Matcha Cheesecake (Serves 6)

Ingredients:

Cheesecake:

16 ounces of Cream Cheese (Room Temperature)

2 Large Eggs (Room Temperature)

2 tablespoons of Heavy Whipping Cream

1/2 cup of Swerve Confectioners

1/2 teaspoon of Vanilla Extract

2 teaspoons of Coconut Flour

1 tablespoon of Matcha Powder

Sugar-Free Maple Syrup (Optional)

Topping:

2 teaspoons of Swerve Confectioners

1/2 cup of Sour Cream

<u>Directions:</u>

1. Add your cream cheese, Swerve, vanilla extract, coconut flour, whipping cream, and matcha powder to your mixing bowl.

2. Mix together until well combined.

3. Add in your eggs one at a time. Pour your cheesecake batter into a well-greased springform pan. You will need a pan that is no larger than 6 to 7 inches so that it fits inside your Instant Pot.

4. Pour 1 1/2 cups water into the bottom of your Instant Pot. Place your steam tray inside with the handles facing up (you will need these later.) Place your cheesecake on top of the tray then lock the lid and make sure that the valve is sealed.

5. Pressure cook on high for 35 minutes then allow a 20 minute natural release.

6. When you open the Instant Pot there may be some water on top of the cheesecake, just gently pat it off with a paper towel. A lot of the times I also find some cracks, but they are easily covered up with the sour cream topping.

7. Mix the sour cream and Swerve together. Spread it out over the top of the cheesecake.

8. Allow your cheesecake to fully cool then store in the refrigerator for several hours before serving. Serve with a drizzle of sugar-free maple syrup.

9. Garnish the top with a sprinkle of matcha powder.

<u>Nutrition Facts:</u>

Calories: 350

Net Carbs: 5.8 grams

Fat: 33.25 grams

Keto Apple Pie (Serves 8)

<u>Ingredients:</u>

<u>Crust:</u>

1 cup of Grass Fed Butter

4 Eggs

1/2 teaspoon of Salt

1 1/2 cups of Coconut Flour

<u>Filling:</u>

6 Macintosh Apples

2 tablespoons of Grass Fed Butter

1/4 cup of Honey

1 tablespoon of Cinnamon

1 teaspoon of Vanilla Extract

Directions:

1. Preheat your oven to 425 degrees.

2. Melt 1 cup of your grass fed butter and combine with eggs and whisk it together.

3. Add your salt and coconut flour.

4. Divide your mixture in half and roll one of your halves into a ball and press and flatten it to your greased 9-inch pie pan.

5. With your other 1/2 of dough, roll and flatten into 1/4 inch of thickness. Place to the side.

6. Peel and slice your apples into desired size pieces.

7. Toss apple pieces, vanilla extract, honey, and cinnamon into a bowl. Make sure apples are all evenly coated in your mixture.

8. Pour your apples into crust lined pan. Place butter on top to allow it to brown and moisten your filling. Cover piece with your rolled out dough that you put to the side. Seal all the edges by pinching them. Slice a few slits on top of your dough so some steam can come out in the oven when cooking.

9. Separate an egg. Whisk the white part. Use a kitchen brush to brush some of the egg on the entire top crust.

10. Place in oven and bake approximately 15 minutes at 425 degrees. Lower to 350 degrees and continue baking for another 40 minutes.

11. Allow it to cool slightly until it is warm.

Nutrition Facts:

Calories: 450

Protein: 8 grams

Fat: 32 grams

Carbs: 27 grams

Keto Caramel (Serves 4)

<u>Ingredients:</u>

1 teaspoon of Erythritol

4 tablespoons of Unsalted Butter

4 tablespoons of Heavy Cream

Pinch of Salt

<u>Directions:</u>

1. Melt your butter in pan and cook until it is golden brown.

2. Pour in heavy cream and combine. Lower your heat and simmer approximately 1 minute.

3. Add in erythritol. Allow to dissolve and add your salt.

4. Cook until it gets stickier and thicker.

5. Pour into your glass container and continue to stir caramel mixture while it cools down and thickens.

<u>Nutrition Facts:</u>

Calories: 163

Fat: 17 grams

Carbs: 0.5 grams

Keto Chocolate & Hazelnut Spread (Serves 6)

Ingredients:

4 tablespoons of Coconut Oil

5 ounces of Hazelnuts

2 tablespoons of Cocoa Powder

1-ounce of Unsalted Butter

1 teaspoon of Vanilla Extract

1 teaspoon of Erythritol (Optional)

Directions:

1. Roast your hazelnuts in a dry and hot frying pan until they turn a nice golden color.

2. Place your nuts in a clean kitchen towel and rub so that some of the shells come off. The shells which are still stuck can stay there.

3. Place your nuts with all the remaining ingredients in a blender or a food processor. Blend to desired consistency. The longer you mix, the smoother the spread.

Nutrition Facts:

Calories: 271

Net Carbs: 2 grams

Keto Chocolate Cheesecake (Serves 8)

<u>Ingredients:</u>

<u>Chocolate Crust:</u>

1 cup of Almond Flour

4 tablespoons of Butter

1/16 teaspoon of Stevia

1 tablespoon of Cocoa Powder

1/2 teaspoon of Cinnamon

Pinch of Salt

<u>Cheesecake Filling:</u>

2 Eggs

16 ounces of Softened Cream Cheese

3/4 cup of Erythritol

1 tablespoon of Cocoa Powder

1/2 cup of Sour Cream

3 ounces of Unsweetened Baker's Chocolate

1 teaspoon of Vanilla Extract

Pinch of Salt

<u>Directions:</u>

1. Preheat your oven to 350 degrees.

2. Melt your butter and combine with cinnamon, almond flour, Stevia, and cocoa powder. Mix together well.

3. Press this crust dough mixture into 9-inch springform pan and bake approximately 15 minutes till crust becomes solid and gets darker.

4. Begin making the cream cheese filling while crust bakes. Beat your erythritol and cream cheese with an electric hand mixer until it is smooth.

5. Add in your vanilla extract, sour cream, eggs, and salt. Beat with mixer until it gets creamy.

6. Melt your baker's chocolate in a small pan over low heat. Stir it constantly.

7. Pour your chocolate and cocoa powder into your cream cheese mixture. Stir with your spatula to combine two mixtures.

8. Pour your cheesecake batter into your pan on top of the crust.

9. Bake for approximately 50 to 60 minutes until your cheesecake sets.

10. Allow it to cool.

11. Run knife around the edges of your pan to loosen cake.

<u>Nutrition Facts:</u>

Calories: 450

Protein: 11 grams

Fat: 40 grams

Carbs: 8 grams

Keto Flan (Serves 4)

Ingredients:

2 Large Eggs

1/8 cup of Water

1 cup of Heavy Whipping Cream

1 tablespoon of Butter

2 Large Egg Yolks

1 tablespoon of Vanilla

1/3 cup Erythritol (For Caramel)

1/4 cup of Erythritol (For Custard)

Directions:

1. In your deep pan, heat up your erythritol for the caramel. Stir it frequently.

2. Add your water and butter.

3. Stir occasionally until your sauce has become a golden brown.

4. Pour into the bottom of each ramekin, covering the bottom nicely. Set to the side and allow them to cool.

5. In your bowl, mix together your heavy whipping cream, remaining erythritol, and vanilla.

6. In a separate bowl, whisk together your whole eggs. Then add in your yolks, whisking once more.

7. Slowly stir your eggs into your cream mix.

8. Pour your custard into each ramekin, on top of the caramel.

9. Place your ramekins into a casserole dish and fill over halfway with hot water. Bake at 350 degrees for 30 minutes. Take your casserole dish out of the oven but leave the ramekins in the hot water for approximately 10 minutes.

10. Using tongs, take out your ramekins and allow them to sit for at least 4 hours, or overnight, in your refrigerator.

11. When ready to eat, take a knife and slowly run it on the inside of the custard to release it from the ramekin.

12. Turn your ramekin upside down and slowly jiggle the custard onto the plate.

Nutrition Facts:

Net Carbs: 2.4 grams

Calories: 298

Keto Hot Chocolate (Serves 1)

Ingredients:

1 cup of Boiling Water

1 ounce Of Unsalted Butter

1/4 teaspoon of Vanilla Extract

1 tablespoon of Cocoa Powder

Directions:

1. Put your ingredients in a tall beaker to use with a hand blender.

2. Mix for approximately 15 to 20 seconds or until there's a fine foam on top.

Nutrition Facts:

Calories: 216

Net Carbs: 1 gram

Keto Ice Cream (Serves 4)

<u>Ingredients:</u>

8 Strawberries

1/2 cup of Heavy Cream

16 drops of EZ-Sweetz

3 ounces of Cream Cheese

1 tablespoon of Lemon Juice

3/4 cup of Ice

1/4 teaspoon of Vanilla Extract

Directions:

1. Place your ingredients in your Vitamix.

2. Using the variable speed setting, start on 1 until the solids are pulverized then rotate to 10 slowly while you use your tamper to push ingredients into blades. Blend together for approximately 30 to 60 seconds until mounds begin to form. Serve immediately or place in the freezer.

Nutrition Facts:

Calories: 179

Protein: 4 grams

Fat: 16 grams

Carbs: 5 grams

Keto Lava Cake (Serves 1)

<u>Ingredients:</u>

1 Medium Egg

1/4 teaspoon of Baking Powder

2 tablespoons of Cocoa Powder

2 tablespoons of Erythritol

1 tablespoon of Heavy Cream

1/2 teaspoon of Vanilla Extract

Pinch of Salt

<u>Directions:</u>

1. Preheat your oven to 350 degrees.

2. Combine your cocoa powder and erythritol. Mix until it is smooth. Remove any clumps that form.

3. In a separate bowl, beat egg till fluffy.

4. Add your heavy cream, vanilla extract, and egg to your cocoa mixture. Add in baking soda and salt.

5. Spray your cooking oil into your mug and pour your batter in. Bake for approximately 10 to 15 minutes at 350 degrees. The top should be set but still jiggly.

6. Allow to relax approximately 3 minutes. Run sharp knife around edges of the ramekin to loosen your cakes.

7. Place your plate upside down onto your mug. Flip mug and plate so mug is now facing upside down on your plate. Tap mug to make your cake gently fall onto your plate.

8. Add your desired optional toppings.

<u>Nutrition Facts:</u>

Calories: 173

Protein: 8 grams

Fat: 13 grams

Carbs: 4 grams

Keto Mug Cookie (Serves 1)

Ingredients:

1 Egg Yolk

1 tablespoon of Butter

1 tablespoon of Erythritol

3 tablespoons of Almond Flour

1 pinch of Cinnamon

1 pinch of Salt

2 tablespoons of Sugar-Free Chocolate Chips

1/8 teaspoon of Vanilla Extract

Directions:

1. Preheat your oven to 350 degrees.

2. Melt your butter in a small-sized pan and allow to brown a bit.

3. Combine your butter with almond flour.

4. Add your cinnamon and erythritol.

5. Add your vanilla extract, egg yolk, and salt.

6. Spray your cup or mug with cooking oil and place in your mixture. Flatten it out to make sure it cooks evenly.

7. Press into your cup.

8. Microwave for 1 minute on high or bake in your oven approximately 10 minutes.

9. Allow it to cool.

<u>Nutritional Facts:</u>

Calories: 330

Protein: 7 grams

Fat: 31 grams

Carbs: 3 grams

Keto Pancakes (Serves 1)

Ingredients:

Pancakes:

3 tablespoons of Coconut Flour

3 Large Egg Whites

1 to 2 tablespoons of Granulated Sweetener

1 tablespoon of Mashed Pumpkin

1/2 teaspoon of Vanilla Extract

1/2 cup of Dairy-Free Milk (More If Necessary)

Pinch of Sea Salt

Pinch of Baking Powder

Coconut Butter Vanilla Glaze:

1 tablespoon of Coconut Butter

1/2 teaspoon of Vanilla Extract

1 tablespoon of Granulated Sweetener

2 tablespoons of Dairy Free Milk

<u>Directions:</u>

1. In your large-sized mixing bowl, sift your coconut flour, sea salt, granulated sweetener, and baking powder to avoid clumps. Mix together well to combine.

2. In your small-sized bowl, whisk your egg whites until stiff peaks form. Add to your dry mixture, along with the mashed pumpkin. Using a tablespoon at a time, add dairy-free milk until a thick batter is formed (you may need more than 1/2 cup). Mix lightly, but do not over mix.

3. Spray your pan with cooking spray and heat on low/medium. Once your pan is hot, pour batter using a 1/4 cup at a time. Cook your pancakes for approximately 2 to 3 minutes or until the edges brown, before flipping very gently and cooking for an extra minute or two, until cooked through. Repeat until all of your pancakes are cooked.

4. To make your coconut butter vanilla glaze, whisk all of your ingredients in a small-sized bowl and top pancakes. Add sprinkles if desired.

Keto Popsicles (Serves 2)

Ingredients:

4 tablespoons of Heavy Cream

2 1/3 tablespoons of Sugar-Free Coconut Milk

4 teaspoons of Sugar-Free Flavored Syrup

Directions:

1. Freeze your Zoku device for approximately 1 day or until completely frozen.

2. Each popsicle will use 4 tablespoons of your total mix. Mix your ingredients and put in the freezer.

3. Bring out your Zoku and place a popsicle stick in it.

4. Add your liquid and wait for approximately 9 minutes.

5. Once completely frozen, screw in your extractor and release mold.

6. Snap on your drip shield.

Nutrition Facts:

Calories: 104

Fat: 10 grams

Carbs: 1 gram

Keto Sansrival (Serves 12)

Ingredients:

Dacquoise:

1/2 cup of Almond Flour

3/4 cup of Egg Whites

1/3 cup of Chopped Roasted Almonds

7/8 cup of Allulose

1 teaspoon of Cream of Tartar

Syrup:

3/4 cup of Allulose

1/4 cup of Water

1/2 cup of Egg Yolks

1 teaspoon Vanilla Bean Paste

French Buttercream:

1 1/2 cups of Softened Cubed Butter

1 cup of Syrup

Directions:

Dacquoise:

1. Preheat your oven to 300 degrees. Line your sheet tray with Silpat or parchment paper.

2. Combine your almond flour and chopped almonds in your bowl. Mix together well until blended. Set to the side.

3. Combine your egg whites and cream of tartar in your mixing bowl.

4. Using a wire attachment, on medium, mix until foamy. Increase the speed then gradually add allulose. Look for medium stiff peaks. Note that because we are not using sugar, the meringue will not whip to stiff peaks.

5. Carefully fold your almond flour and chopped almonds mixture into the meringue until homogeneous.

6. Evenly distribute your mixture into three-ring molds or pipe into three 8" rounds. Even the surface using an offset spatula.

7. Bake in the center of the oven for approximately 30 minutes or until golden. Cool and set to the side. Note that this may be made ahead of time. To store, wrap in plastic wrap and refrigerate.

Syrup:

1. In a heavy-bottomed saucepan, combine your water and allulose.

2. Set up a candy thermometer, if using. Set the saucepan over a low heat and allow it to cook to soft ball stage or 240 degrees.

3. Meantime, while your syrup is cooking, combine your egg yolks and vanilla paste in a bowl.

4. Using a wire whisk, whip on high until light and doubled in volume, approximately 8 minutes.

5. When your syrup reaches 240 degrees, remove from heat. Reduce your mixer speed to low. In a slow, even stream, away from the whisk, gently pour in your syrup. Continue until all your syrup has been added.

6. Transfer to another container and allow it to cool. Note that this may be made ahead of time. To store, refrigerate in an airtight container.

French Buttercream:

1. Place the butter in your mixing bowl. Using a paddle attachment, cream your butter at low speed until soft. Occasionally scrape the bottom and sides of the bowl. Increase the speed to medium and continue to whip until volume increases.

2. Turn your mixer off. Add your syrup and, on low speed, continue to mix until the buttercream is light and smooth.

Assemble:

1. Layer your dacquoise and buttercream alternately.

2. Frost the entire cake with the buttercream and garnish with chopped almonds.

Nutrition Facts:

Calories: 348

Net Carbs: 5 grams

Protein: 7 grams

Keto Skillet Brownies (Serves 4)

<u>Ingredients:</u>

<u>Brownies:</u>

1 Egg

1/2 teaspoon of Baking Powder

6 tablespoons of Butter

1/3 cup of Erythritol

1/4 cup of Almond Flour

1/2 teaspoon of Vanilla Extract

1/3 cup of Cocoa Powder

1/4 cup of Walnuts

Pinch of Salt

<u>*Peanut Butter Drizzle:*</u>

1 tablespoon of Peanut butter

1 tablespoon of Butter

Directions:

1. Preheat your oven to 350 degrees.

2. Melt your butter in a small-sized pan and add in your erythritol. Allow to dissolve.

3. Pour your mixture into a mixing bowl and add in your salt, vanilla extract, and cocoa powder.

4. Add in your egg and beat until it is well combined.

5. Add your baking powder and almond flour.

6. Fold in your choice of nuts. I used walnuts.

7. Pour brownie batter into your 6-inch cast iron skillet.

8. Place in your oven and bake for approximately 30 minutes. The top will be set but still jiggly.

9. Add peanut butter drizzle if you desire.

<u>**Nutrition Facts:**</u>

Calories: 333

Protein: 6 grams

Fat: 32 grams

Carbs: 3 grams

Keto Strawberry Cheesecake (Serves 8)

Ingredients:

Crust:

2 tablespoons of Splenda

4 tablespoons of Butter

3/4 cup of Pecans

3/4 cup of Almond Flour

Filling:

9 Strawberries

4 Eggs

1/2 tablespoon of Lemon Juice

1 1/2 pounds of Cream Cheese

1/2 tablespoon of Liquid Vanilla

1/2 teaspoon of EZ-Sweetz

1/4 cup of Sour Cream

<u>Directions:</u>

1. Preheat your oven to approximately 400 degrees.

2. Crush up your pecans.

3. In your small-sized saucepan, melt your butter and add in your almond flour, pecans, and Splenda.

4. Mix crust in your saucepan for several minutes until your ingredients are combined.

5. Grease 9-inch springform pan. Line the bottom with your crust mixture.

6. Cook at 400 degrees approximately 7 minutes until your crust begins to brown.

7. Combine all your filling ingredients in a stand mixer and combine well.

8. Slice some additional strawberries and line side of crust if you'd like.

9. Add your filling on top of your crust.

10. Top with more strawberries if you'd like.

11. Put cheesecake in your oven and drop it from 400 degrees to 250 degrees as soon as it's in the oven.

12. Cook for approximately 60 to 90 minutes until your cheesecake has set.

13. Allow it to cool.

<u>Nutrition Facts:</u>

Calories: 535

Protein: 13 grams

Fat: 49 grams

Carbs: 9 grams

Keto Truffles (Serves 12)

Ingredients:

1/2 cup of Organic Heavy Cream

2 tablespoons of Honey

1 cup of Organic Dark Chocolate

2 tablespoons of Raw Cocoa Powder

2 tablespoons of Grass Fed Butter

1/2 teaspoon of Pure Vanilla Extract

1/2 teaspoon of Cinnamon

Pinch of Sea Salt

Directions:

1. Heat cream over a low flame. Don't allow it to boil.

2. Chop your chocolate into small-sized pieces.

3. When simmering add in your chocolate and stir until it is combined with cream. Add in your butter and stir in until it is melted completely.

4. Turn off heat and add your cinnamon, vanilla, honey, and salt. Mix well to combine.

5. Place in refrigerator for approximately 1 hour. Stir every 20 minutes.

6. Once cooled and hardened, scoop some of your mixture out and roll into small balls about 1 1/2 inches in diameter.

7. Place each truffle ball on a baking sheet lined with parchment paper and refrigerate approximately 30 minutes.

8. Roll in hands to smooth balls out. Place your cocoa powder in a bowl and add your truffles. Shake and roll them in your cocoa powder to coat evenly.

Nutrition Facts:

Calories: 142

Fat: 12 grams

Carbs: 6 grams

Keto Vanilla Custard (Serves 4)

Ingredients:

6 Egg Yolks

1 teaspoon of Vanilla Extract

1/2 cup of Unsweetened Almond Milk

4 tablespoons of Melted Coconut Oil or Unsalted Butter

1 teaspoon of Erythritol (Optional)

Directions:

1. Whisk together your egg yolks, almond milk, vanilla, and optional sweetener in a medium metal bowl.

2. Slowly mix in your melted coconut oil or butter. Be sure the oil isn't too hot, or the eggs may cook unevenly.

3. Place your bowl over a saucepan of simmering water. Whisk your mixture constantly and vigorously until thickened. Your instant-read thermometer should register 140 degrees for 3 full minutes. Usually, this means about 5 minutes of total cooking time.

4. Remove your custard from the water bath. Serve either warm or chilled.

Nutrition Facts:

Calories: 215

Net Carbs: 1 gram

Key Lime Cheesecake In A Jar (Serves 8)

Ingredients:

Stabilized Whipped Cream:

1 cup of Heavy Whipping Cream

4 teaspoons of Cold Water

1 teaspoon of Grass-Fed Gelatin

2 tablespoons of Low-Carb Sweetener (Powdered)

Crust:

1/2 teaspoon of Cinnamon

3/4 cup + 2 tablespoons of Almond Flour

4 tablespoons of Melted Unsalted Butter

1 1/2 tablespoons of Low-Carb Sweetener

<u>*Filling:*</u>

1/4 cup of Low-Carb Sweetener

12 ounces of Softened Cream Cheese

1/2 teaspoon of Vanilla Extract

Juice from 4 Key Limes

Zest of 2 Key Limes

Directions:

<u>*Crust:*</u>

1. In your small-sized bowl, combine your cinnamon, almond flour, and sweetener.

2. Add your melted butter then divide between eight 4-ounce jars.

3. Press down to form the crust at bottom of each cup.

<u>*Stabilized Whipped Cream:*</u>

1. In your small-sized pan, combine your gelatin and cold water. Allow it to stand to soften your gelatin.

2. Place over a low heat, stirring constantly, until your gelatin dissolves.

3. Remove from your heat. Allow it to cool slightly at room temperature (do not allow it to set).

4. Whip the cream with your icing sugar, until slightly thick.

5. While slowly beating, stream in your gelatin liquid to the whipping cream.

6. Whip at high speed until stiff. Set to the side.

Filling:

1. In your medium-sized bowl, blend all of your filling ingredients with an electric mixer until well combined.

2. Fold in half of the stabilized whipped cream.

3. Pipe or spoon your filling over crust in each jar, dividing evenly between your jars.

4. Top off each jar with your remaining whipped cream.

5. Decorate with your additional lime zest and slices.

Nutrition Facts:

Calories: 377

Net Carbs: 2.7 grams

Lemon Bar Fat Bombs (Serves 30)

Ingredients:

1/2 cup of Coconut Butter

1/4 cup of Coconut Flour

1 cup of Melted Coconut Oil

2 cups of Raw Cashews (Boiled for 12 minutes or Soaked for 2 Hours)

1/3 cup of Shredded Coconut

1/16 teaspoon of Pink Himalayan Salt

1/8 teaspoon of Powdered Stevia

Zest of 1 Large Lemon

Juice of 2 Large Lemons

Directions:

1. Combine all of your ingredients in a food processor and blend until well-combined.

2. Transfer your mixture to medium-sized bowl and place in your freezer for 20 to 30 minutes to cool (they may take slightly longer if you chose to boil the cashews rather than soak).

3. Remove your mixture from the freezer and form into balls.

4. Place your balls in your freezer for 20 minutes to harden. I recommend putting them on a cookie sheet or plate lined with parchment paper to avoid the bottoms sticking.

5. Remove from freezer once solid. Store in an airtight container in your refrigerator or freezer.

Nutrition Facts:

Fat: 15 grams

Calories: 165

Lemon Blueberry Shortbread Cookies (Serves 9)

Ingredients:

Blueberry Glaze:

1/4 cup of Coconut Oil

1/4 cup of Blueberries

2 tablespoons of Sukrin Melis

Cookies:

1 Egg

1 tablespoon of Lemon Juice

1/2 cup of Sukrin Sweetener

1/2 teaspoon of Baking Powder

1 Egg Yolk

1 teaspoon of Vanilla Extract

1/4 cup of Softened Butter

3/4 cup of Sifted Almond Flour

1 tablespoon of Coconut Flour

1/2 teaspoon of Salt

1/2 teaspoon of Xanthan Gum

Directions:

1. Preheat your oven to 350 degrees.

2. Beat together your butter and Sukrin until it is creamy.

3. Add in your egg yolk and egg along with your vanilla and lemon juice. Mix it together well.

4. In a separate bowl, sift your almond flour and combine with the rest of dry ingredients excluding your xanthan gum.

5. Slowly pour your dry ingredients into wet ingredients, beating your mixture the entire time.

6. When combined add your xanthan gum and mix it together well.

7. Line your baking sheet using parchment paper and measure out even-sized cookie dough balls. Flatten each one and ensure each one cooks evenly.

8. Bake approximately 8 to 10 minutes.

9. Allow it to cool completely.

10. Make your glaze. Combine all of your ingredients in your immersion blender.

11. Allow glaze to sit and thicken up. Put a teaspoon of glaze over each of your cookies.

12. Refrigerate your glazed cookies for approximately an hour.

<u>Nutrition Facts:</u>

Calories: 170

Protein: 3 grams

Lemon Cheesecake Fat Bombs (Serves 12)

Ingredients:

1/4 cup of Melted Coconut Oil

1 tablespoon of Finely Grated Lemon Zest

4 tablespoons of Softened Unsalted Butter

4 ounces of Softened Cream Cheese

1 teaspoon of Lemon Juice

Stevia

Lemon Extract (Optional)

Directions:

1. Blend all of your ingredients with your hand mixer until smooth.

2. Pour into your cupcake liners, tins, or molds.

3. Freeze until firm. At least a few hours, preferably overnight.

4. Sprinkle with your lemon zest.

<u>Nutrition Facts:</u>

Calories: 106

Net Carbs: 0.25 grams

Lemon Cupcakes w/ Raspberry Frosting (Serves 12)

<u>Ingredients:</u>

<u>Lemon Cupcakes:</u>

2 1/3 cups of Almond Flour

1/2 teaspoon of Xanthan Gum

1 teaspoon of Baking Powder

2 teaspoons of Lemon Extract

3/4 cup of Granulated Stevia/Erythritol Blend

1/2 teaspoon of Sea Salt

2 tablespoons of Melted Butter

2 tablespoons of Lemon Zest

3/4 cup of Unsweetened Almond Milk

3 Large Eggs

1 tablespoon of Vanilla Extract

Raspberry Frosting:

16 ounces of Softened Cream Cheese

1/3 cup of Granulated Stevia/Erythritol Blend

2 tablespoons of Softened Butter

3 tablespoons of Whipping Cream

3/4 cup of Unsweetened Frozen Raspberries

1 teaspoon of Lemon Juice

1 teaspoon of Vanilla Extract

Directions:

1. Preheat oven to 350 degrees and line your cupcake pan with papers.

2. In your large-sized bowl, whisk together your almond flour, baking powder, salt, xanthan gum, sweetener, and zest until combined.

3. Whisk your melted butter into the dry ingredients. The mixture should form into coarse crumbs.

4. Add your eggs and stir until incorporated. The batter will begin to stick together.

5. Add your almond milk, vanilla, and lemon extract and whisk until the batter is smooth.

6. Carefully fill the prepared cupcake papers until they are about 3/4 full—about 2 heaping tablespoons for each cupcake.

7. Place your cupcakes in a preheated oven and bake for approximately 29 to 32 minutes or until the cupcake bounces back when pressed.

8. Allow your cupcakes to cool on a rack until they reach room temperature before frosting.

9. In your large-sized bowl, whip together your cream cheese and butter using an electric mixer.

10. Blend in your sweetener and frozen raspberries until combined.

11. Add your whipping cream, lemon juice, and vanilla and blend until smooth.

12. Using a piping bag, frost cupcakes as desired.

<u>Nutrition Facts:</u>

Calories: 336

Net Carbs: 5.75 grams

Fat: 30.5 grams

Low-Carb Trifle (Serves 4)

Ingredients:

1 Ripe Avocado

3/4 cup of Coconut Cream

1/2 Ripe Banana

1 tablespoon of Vanilla Extract

2 ounces of Roasted Pecans

3 ounces of Fresh Raspberries

1 tablespoon of Lime Juice

Zest of Lime Juice

Directions:

1. Mix your banana, avocado, lime, coconut cream, and half of your vanilla in a small-sized bowl using an immersion blender or your a fork.

2. Mix your berries with the remaining vanilla in your separate bowl.

3. Fill glasses or dessert bowls with alternating layers of the two mixtures.

4. Place your frying pan over a medium-high heat and add your nuts. Roast until golden brown. Stir frequently to avoid burning.

5. Top your dessert with roasted nuts.

Nutrition Facts:

Calories: 368

Net Carbs: 8 grams

Macadamia & Speculoos Biscotti (Serves 10)

Ingredients:

2 Large Eggs

3 ounces of Swerve Confectioners

7 ounces of Superfine Almond Flour

1 teaspoon of Xanthan Gum

1 teaspoon of Baking Powder

2 1/2 ounces of Dry Roasted Macadamia Nuts

1 teaspoon of Vanilla Bean Paste

2 ounces of Melted Salted Butter

1 tablespoon of Speculoos Spice Blend

Directions:

1. Preheat your oven to 325 degrees. In your bowl, combine your almond flour, sweetener, baking powder, xanthan gum, vanilla paste, macadamia, and spice blend. Mix together well.

2. In your separate bowl, melt your butter. Add your eggs. Beat well.

3. Add your butter and egg mixture to the dry ingredients.

4. Mix well and form into a dough.

5. Transfer your dough to a work surface, pat, and form into an even, flattened, oblong or square-ish shaped log. Note that the dough is sticky. To help with the shaping, dust hands with almond flour.

6. Transfer your dough to a parchment lined sheet tray and bake for approximately 30 minutes or until firm, lightly golden, and top is slightly cracked. Remove from your oven. Set to the side to cool, approximately 15 minutes.

7. When cool, slice your loaf into half inch thick slices.

8. Preheat your oven to 250 degrees.

9. Line slices on a parchment lined sheet tray. Bake for approximately 15 minutes. Flip your slices and bake for another 15 minutes.

10. Turn your oven off. Allow the the biscotti to cool in your oven until crisp, crunchy, and dry. Store in an airtight container.

<u>Nutrition Facts:</u>

Calories: 190

Net Carbs: 2.7 grams

Macaroon Fat Bombs (Serves 10)

Ingredients:

1/4 cup of Organic Almond Flour

1/2 cup of Shredded Coconut

2 tablespoons of Swerve

3 Egg Whites

1 tablespoon of Vanilla Extract

1 tablespoon of Coconut Oil

Directions:

1. In your bowl mix almond flour, coconut, and swerve until well blended.

2. Melt your coconut oil in a small-sized saucepan and add your vanilla extract to it.

3. In the meantime, chill your medium-sized bowl in your freezer for mounting the egg whites.

4. Add your melted coconut oil to the flour mix and blend well.

5. Put your egg whites in your chilled bowl and whisk until stiff, very foamy holding stiff peaks.

6. Incorporate your egg whites into your flour mix, trying to not over mix and to preserve some of the volume from the eggs whites.

7. Spoon your mixture onto a cookie sheet, or into muffin cups.

8. Bake at 400 degrees for 8 minutes or until macaroons start to brown on top.

9. Remove from your oven and allow it to cool before removing from the cookie sheet.

Nutrition Facts:

Calories: 46

Net Carbs: 0.5 grams

Matcha Skillet Souffle (Serves 1)

Ingredients:

3 Large Eggs

7 Whole Raspberries

1 tablespoon of Butter

1 tablespoon of Unsweetened Cocoa Powder

1 tablespoon of Matcha Powder

1 teaspoon of Vanilla Extract

2 tablespoons of Swerve Confectioners

1/4 cup of Whipped Cream

1 tablespoon of Coconut Oil

Directions:

1. Set your oven to broil, and preheat a cast iron pan over a medium heat. Separate your eggs into yolks and whites.

2. Whip your whites with 1 tablespoon of Swerve confectioners. Once peaks form add in your matcha powder Continue to whip until the peaks become stiff. (I've also done this by adding everything at once to a stand mixer, but it failed to whip with a hand mixer.)

3. Use a fork to break up the yolks. Mix in the vanilla then add a small amount of the whipped whites. Carefully fold the rest of the whites into your yolk mixture.

4. Add your tablespoon of butter to the cast iron pan. Allow it to melt then add the souffle mixture to the pan. Turn the heat to low then place the raspberries on top. Allow it to cook until your eggs puff up and feel set if you carefully tap the top.

5. Move your skillet to the oven and watch it carefully. Remove once the top starts to brown. If you leave it in too long it may turn quite dark or burn.

6. Melt your coconut oil then whisk in your cocoa powder and remaining tablespoon of Swerve confectioners. Drizzle across the top. Serve with 1/4 cup of whipped cream.

<u>Nutrition Facts:</u>

Calories: 578

Net Carbs: 5 grams

Fat: 51 grams

Mexican Chocolate Pudding (Serves 2)

<u>Ingredients:</u>

1 tablespoon of Coconut Milk

1 teaspoon of Ceylon Cinnamon

1 Avocado

2 1/2 tablespoons of Raw Cocoa Powder

1 tablespoon of Coconut Milk

1/16 teaspoon of Ground Cayenne Pepper

1/2 teaspoon of Pure Vanilla Extract

1 tablespoon of Sweetener

Pinch of Stevia

Pinch of Pink Himalayan Sea Salt

Directions:

1. Cut and pit your avocado. Blend in food processor until smooth.

2. Add your coconut milk, vanilla extract, and cocoa powder. Blend it until it is smooth.

3. Add your cinnamon, sweetener, ground cayenne pepper, and Stevia.

4. Blend until smooth. Get rid of all your chunks.

5. Sprinkle with sea salt.

Nutrition Facts:

Calories: 180

Protein: 3 grams

Fat: 15 grams

Carbs: 3.5 grams

Mini Cheesecakes (Serves 8)

<u>Ingredients:</u>

<u>*Cheesecake:*</u>

1 Egg

1/4 cup of Erythritol

8 ounces of Cream Cheese

1/2 teaspoon of Vanilla Extract

1/2 teaspoon of Lemon Juice

Pinch of Salt

<u>*Crust:*</u>

1/2 cup of Almond Meal

2 tablespoons of Butter

<u>Directions:</u>

1. Preheat your oven to 350 degrees.

2. To make your crust, melt your butter until it is liquid and then mix with your almond meal.

3. Take a teaspoon of dough at a time and press into bottom of your muffin tin. You can line your pan with cupcake liners to make removal easy.

4. Bake your crusts approximately 5 minutes at 350 degrees. Should be crispy and slightly brown.

5. Beat your cream cheese with your electric hand mixer until it is creamy. Add in lemon, vanilla extract, erythritol, and egg. Beat until well combined.

6. Fill all the crust bottomed muffin tin cups. Do so evenly and nearly to the top.

7. Bake for approximately 15 minutes at 350 degrees. Cheesecakes should be a little jiggly.

8. Allow it to cool.

9. Slide knife around outer edges of each cup to loosen.

<u>Nutrition Facts:</u>

Calories: 176

Protein: 4 grams

Fat: 16 grams

Carbs: 2 grams

Mint Chocolate Chip Ice Cream (Serves 4)

<u>Ingredients:</u>

1 cup of Heavy Cream

1/2 teaspoon of Liquid Stevia Extract

1/2 cup of Light Cream

1 Square Dark Chocolate (Optional)

1/2 teaspoon of Vanilla (Optional)

Several drops of Peppermint Extract (Optional)

Several drops of Green Food Coloring (Optional)

<u>Directions:</u>

1. Place your ice cream bowl in your freezer 4 to 12 hours ahead of time.

2. Place all of your ingredients in ice cream bowl except the chocolate.

3. Whisk together well.

4. Place in your freezer for approximately 5 minutes.

5. Set up your ice cream maker and add in liquid.

6. Make ice cream according to your machine's instructions. A few minutes before ice cream sets, add in your chocolate shavings.

7. Store in air tight container and place back in the freezer.

8. Allow to freeze.

Nutrition Facts:

Calories: 295

Fat: 31 grams

Carbs: 3.5 grams

Mocha Peppermint Fat Bombs (Serves 16)

Ingredients:

3/4 cup of Melted Coconut Butter

3 tablespoons of Melted Coconut Oil

1/4 teaspoon of Peppermint Extract

3 tablespoons of Hemp Seeds

2 teaspoons of Instant Coffee Powder

2 tablespoons of Organic Cocoa Powder

5 to 8 drops of Liquid Stevia

Directions:

1. Mix together your melted coconut butter, 1 tablespoon of coconut oil, hemp seeds, and peppermint extract.

2. Pour into molds about 3/4 of the way.

3. Refrigerate until firm.

4. Stir together 2 tablespoons of melted coconut oil, cocoa powder, instant coffee, and stevia.

5. Drizzle on top of your fat bombs.

6. Refrigerate again until completely hardened.

7. Pop out of your molds and transfer to an airtight container.

8. Store in your refrigerator or freezer.

<u>Nutrition Facts:</u>

Carbs: 4 grams

Calories: 121

No Bake Lemon Cheesecake

<u>Ingredients:</u>

8 ounces of Softened Cream Cheese

2 ounces of Heavy Cream

1 teaspoon of Stevia Glycerite

1 tablespoon of Lemon Juice

1 teaspoon of Vanilla Flavoring

1 teaspoon of Splenda

<u>Directions:</u>

1. Mix all your ingredients together and then whip it into a pudding-like consistency. Spoon mixture into small serving cups and then refrigerate till it sets.

No Flour Chocolate Cake (Serves 8)

Ingredients:

3 Eggs

1 cup of Swerve Erythritol (separated into 1/2 cup, 1/4 cup, 1/4 cup)

1/2 cup of Cocoa Powder

1/2 cup of Butter

4 ounces of Unsweetened Baker's Chocolate

1/2 teaspoon of Salt

1 teaspoon of Vanilla Extract

Directions:

1. Preheat your oven to 300 degrees. Set up your double boiler to melt your butter and baker's chocolate together. If no boiler use your pan over a low heat.

2. Once they are both melted, combine them both together. Add in 1/2 cup of erythritol and stir well over a low flame until it is dissolved.

3. Separate 3 eggs and beat your eggs whites until foamy. Add 1/4 cup of erythritol slowly while beating your egg whites. Should form stiff peaks and turn glossy.

4. Clean your beaters and beat your 3 egg yolks. Slowly add in the last 1/4 cup of erythritol. Yolks should turn pale yellow and double in volume.

5. Add your chocolate mixture to egg yolks. Stir well.

6. Add your cocoa powder. Stir well. Add your salt and vanilla.

7. Add a third of your egg whites and fold in gently. Repeat this process until all your eggs whites have been added and folded in.

8. Spray your springform pan with cooking oil. Pour in your chocolate batter. Bake for approximately 35 minutes.

9. Dust with powdered erythritol.

<u>Nutrition Facts:</u>

Calories: 240

Carbs: 2 grams

Fat: 21 grams

Nutella Brownies (Serves 4)

Ingredients:

4 Eggs

4 tablespoons of Erythritol

1 Cup of Nutella

Directions:

1. Preheat your oven to 350 degrees.

2. Place your Nutella in a microwave for approximately 15-second intervals, stirring until it gets really soft.

3. Crack your eggs and mix with electric mixer until they've tripled in volume and become a lighter yellow color. Should take approximately 5 to 8 minutes.

4. Combine your Nutella and eggs. Whisk until it is combined. Add your erythritol.

5. Add your mixture to ramekins. Put your ramekins on a cookie sheet. Bake for approximately 25 to 30 minutes.

6. Allow it to cool.

Nutrition Facts:

Calories: 396

Protein: 12 grams

Fat: 35 grams

Carbs: 4 grams

Nutella Sundae (Serves 2)

Ingredients:

4 scoops of Low-Carb Ice Cream

2 tablespoons of Homemade Nutella

2 Strawberries

Sprinkles

Whipped Cream

Directions:

1. Mix it all together.

2. Place in your bowl.

3. Add your toppings.

<u>**Nutrition Facts:**</u>

Calories: 191

Protein: 4 grams

Fat: 14 grams

Carbs: 10 grams

Nutty Coconut Fat Bombs (Serves 15)

Ingredients:

1 1/2 cups of Walnuts

2 tablespoons of Almond Butter

1/4 cup of Coconut Butter + 1 tablespoon

1/2 cup of Shredded Coconut

2 tablespoons of Chia Seeds

2 tablespoons of Flax Meal

1/2 teaspoon of Vanilla Bean Powder

2 tablespoons of Hemp Seeds

2 tablespoons of Cacao Nibs

1 teaspoon of Cinnamon

1/4 teaspoon of Kosher Salt

Chocolate Drizzle:

1/2 teaspoon of Coconut Oil

1 ounce of Bittersweet or Unsweetened Chocolate (Chopped)

Directions:

1. In the bowl of your food processor, combine all of your ingredients except for the cacao nibs. Pulse for about 1 to 2 minutes, until the mixture starts to break down. It will first become powdery and will stick together, but still be crumbly.

2. Keep processing until the oils start to release a bit and the mixture sticks together easily - just be careful not to over process or you'll have nut butter. If your mixture seems dry and if you're not using the maple syrup, you may need the extra tablespoon of coconut butter to help it come together. Once your mixture is sticking together well, pulse in your cacao nibs to incorporate them.

3. Use a small-sized cookie scoop or a tablespoon scoop to divide the mixture into equal pieces. Use your hands to roll into balls and place on a plate.

4. If desired, make your chocolate drizzle by melting the chocolate and coconut oil together in your microwave for 30 seconds to 1 minute, or until it's completely melted. Drizzle over the balls and place in the refrigerator or freezer to firm up.

5. Store in an airtight container zip-top bag in the refrigerator or freezer.

Nutrition Facts:

Calories: 164

Fat: 14 grams

Panna Cotta & Cream Hearts (Serves 8)

<u>Ingredients:</u>

<u>Panna Cotta:</u>

2 cups of Organic Heavy Whipping Cream

2 teaspoons of Gelatin

2 tablespoons of Swerve

1 tablespoon of Vanilla Extract

<u>Cream:</u>

2 cups of Organic Heavy Whipping Cream

2 teaspoons of Gelatin

6 Organic or Pastured Egg Yolks

4 tablespoons of Swerve

1 tablespoon of Vanilla Extract

1 teaspoon of Butter (For Greasing)

Zest of 1 Organic Lemon

Decoration:

2 tablespoons of Chopped Roasted Hazelnuts

Directions:

Panna Cotta:

1. Sprinkle your gelatin on the cream and stir well.

2. In your small-sized saucepan warm the cream on a low flame stirring constantly until all the gelatin is dissolved.

3. Add your Swerve and vanilla extract and keep stirring for another minute. Do not let the cream come to a boil. After a minute turn off your flame and allow it to sit for about a minute.

4. Grease your springform with your butter.

5. Pour half of your panna cotta mixture in the bottom of your springform and allow it to cool.

6. Keep the remaining panna cotta fluid by keeping it in a warm oven (170 degrees).

<u>Cream:</u>

1. Mix your cream and gelatin and stir together well.

2. In the same small-sized saucepan start warming the cream on a low flame.

3. In your medium-sized bowl, whisk your egg yolks with Swerve and your lemon zest until they are well-emulsified (they should be whitish and fluffy).

4. Slowly add a cup of warm cream to your egg mixture, whisking the whole time and being careful not to get lumps.

5. Once your mix is fluid and blended with the cup of cream add it to your saucepan carefully, constantly whisking.

6. Bring your mix to a simmer, keep whisking, and cook for approximately 3 minutes, until your cream starts to thicken.

7. Allow it to cool for approximately 5 minutes, whisking occasionally.

8. Once your panna cotta layer has solidified at the top, pour your cooled cream into your springform pan distributing it evenly, the cream should be pretty thick and solid but still spreadable.

9. Pour the last half of your panna cotta on top and allow it to cool.

10. Once cooled to room temperature you can put your springform in the refrigerator for 3 hours or overnight.

11. Remove border from your springform after loosening the sides with a pointed knife.

12. Cut as many hearts as possible into your panna cotta and cream.

13. Remove the hearts with a flat spatula and a knife, cutting off the extra dough.

14. Serve cold with a sprinkle of toasted hazelnuts.

Nutrition Facts:

Calories: 467

Fat: 53 grams

Peanut Butter Chocolate Truffles

Ingredients:

6 ounces of Sugar-Free Chocolate

1 1/2 cups of Powdered Erythritol

4 tablespoons of Melted Butter

1 cup of Peanut Butter

Directions:

1. Melt your butter.

2. Mix your peanut butter, powdered erythritol, and melted butter together.

3. Scoop out your 2 tablespoons of mixture and roll out into small-sized balls. Lay on your baking sheet lined with parchment paper. Chill in your refrigerator for approximately 30 minutes.

4. Melt your chocolate in a small-sized bowl for approximately 10 to 20 seconds in your microwave. Stir it well.

5. Place one of your truffles in your bowl at a time and rotate it with a spoon so that chocolate covers every side. Take out and allow excess chocolate to fall off.

6. Place back on your baking sheet lined with parchment paper and place in refrigerator for another hour to chill.

Nutrition Facts:

Calories: 200

Carbs: 5 grams

Protein: 6 grams

Fat: 17 grams

Peanut Butter Cookies (Serves 15)

Ingredients:

1 Egg

1 cup of Peanut Butter

1/2 cup of Powdered Erythritol

Directions:

1. Preheat your oven to 350 degrees.

2. Combine your ingredients and mix well.

3. Roll your mix into 1-inch balls and place on a baking sheet lined with parchment paper.

4. Bake for approximately 10 to 15 minutes till cookie edges begin to turn dark brown.

5. Allow it to cool on a wire rack.

Nutrition Facts:

Calories: 105

Protein: 4 grams

Fat: 9 grams

Carbs: 2 grams

Peanut Butter Fluff Fat Bombs (Serves 8)

Ingredients:

1/2 cup of Heavy Whipping Cream

5 tablespoons of Swerve Confectioners

2 1/4 tablespoons of Natural Peanut Butter

1/2 square of Unsweetened Chocolate or Lily's Chocolate Chips

4 ounces of Softened Cream Cheese

1/2 teaspoon of Vanilla

Directions:

1. In your medium-sized bowl, beat your heavy whipping cream until it almost doubles in size.

2. In a separate bowl, add your softened cream cheese, natural peanut butter, swerve, and vanilla then beat with your mixer until the fluff is smooth and creamy.

3. Combine the two and mix on low until thoroughly combined and smooth.

4. Grate your unsweetened chocolate shavings on top or add Lily's Chocolate Chips to fluff.

5. Best if kept in the refrigerator overnight and served the next day.

Nutrition Facts:

Fat: 13.4 grams

Net Carbs: 1.7 grams

Pina Colada Fat Bombs (Serves 16)

Ingredients:

2 teaspoons of Pineapple Essence

1 teaspoon of Rum Essence

1/2 cup of Coconut Cream

1/2 cup of Boiling Water

2 tablespoons of Gelatin

3 teaspoons of Erythritol

Directions:

1. Dissolve your gelatin and erythritol in your boiling water in a heatproof jug and add your pineapple essence.

2. Allow it to cool for 5 minutes.

3. Add your coconut cream and rum extract and continue stirring for 2 minutes.

4. Pour into silicon molds and set for at least 1 hour, depending on the size of your mold.

5. Gently remove from your mold. Store in the refrigerator.

Nutrition Facts:

Calories: 23

Fat: 2 grams

Carbs: 0.4 grams

Pink Lemonade Cloud Cake (Serves 2)

Ingredients:

Layers:

1/4 teaspoon of Powdered Stevia

1 Oopsie Roll

Frosting:

2 tablespoons of Erythritol

2 Strawberries

1/3 cup of Softened Butter

1 teaspoon of Lemon Zest

1/2 teaspoon of Poppy Seeds

1 teaspoon of Fresh Lemon Juice

1 tablespoon of Heavy Cream

Pinch of Salt

Directions:

1. Make your oopsie rolls. If you want them to be sweeter add some Stevia to your batter while making them.

2. Once cooked and you've allowed to cool, use a mug to stamp out uniformly sized circles of your oopsie rolls.

3. Once the layers are ready, beat your erythritol and butter until it is creamy. Add a tablespoon of your cream, lemon zest, and lemon juice.

4. Add poppy seeds and finely chopped strawberries.

5. Place frosting mixture into Ziploc bag and remove as much air as possible before twisting the bag and snipping the top.

6. Lay an oopsie roll on your plate and frost the outside of the cake. Follow up by filling in the middle.

7. Stack another oopsie roll on top of the frosted oopsie roll and gently press down. Repeat the previous step. Do this until you have 3 layers of oopsie rolls.

8. Garnish with frosting and your walnut.

9. Chill in your refrigerator for approximately 1 hour.

Nutrition Facts:

Calories: 430

Fat: 42 grams

Carbs: 3 grams

Pumpkin Maple Flaxseed Muffins   (Serves 10)

Ingredients:

1 Egg

1/3 cup of Erythritol

1 cup of Pure Pumpkin Puree

1 1/4 cups of Ground Flax Seeds

1/2 tablespoon of Baking Powder

1 tablespoon of Cinnamon

1/2 teaspoon of Vanilla Extract

1/2 teaspoon of Salt

1/4 cup of Walden Farm's Maple Syrup

1 tablespoon of Pumpkin Pie Spice

1/2 teaspoon of Apple Cider Vinegar

2 tablespoons of Coconut Oil

<u>**Directions:**</u>

1. Add your cupcake liners to your muffin tin. Preheat your oven to 350 degrees.

2. Grind your flax seeds for 1 second in your Nutribullet.

3. Combine your dry ingredients and stir well to disperse evenly.

4. Add your pumpkin puree. Mix well.

5. Add your vanilla extract, maple syrup, and pumpkin spice.

6. Add your coconut oil, apple cider vinegar mix, and egg. Mix well.

7. Add a large tablespoon of mixture to each muffin liner and top with pumpkin seeds. Allow some room for muffins to rise.

8. Bake for approximately 20 minutes. Tops should brown slightly.

9. Allow it to cool. Add any toppings or butter to muffins.

<u>Nutrition Facts:</u>

Calories: 120

Fat: 8.4 grams

Carbs: 2.2 grams

Pumpkin Pecan Tart (Serves 2)

<u>Ingredients:</u>

<u>*Crust:*</u>

1 teaspoon of Cinnamon

2 tablespoons of Melted Butter

1/2 cup of Almond Flour

Pinch of Salt

<u>*Filling:*</u>

1/2 cup of Pumpkin Puree

1/2 teaspoon of Vanilla Extract

1/2 cup of Ricotta Cheese

1/4 teaspoon of Pumpkin Pie Spice

1 teaspoon of Cinnamon

1 Egg White

2 tablespoons of Erythritol

1 Egg

Pinch of Salt

Topping:

16 Pecans

Sugar-Free Maple Syrup

Directions:

1. Preheat your oven to 350 degrees. Combine crust ingredients in a bowl.

2. Mix well and press into your mini tartlet pans. I used 4 1/2 inch pans. Let your tart crusts bake in oven approximately 10 minutes. Let cool while you work on the filling.

3. Combine your egg, egg white, pumpkin puree, and ricotta cheese.

4. Mix in the rest of the filling ingredients. Stir well to combine.

5. Once crusts are cooled, pour your filling onto your crusts. Place tart pans on baking sheet and bake approximately 20 minutes.

6. Remove from oven and add pecans to top. Place back in your oven approximately 10 minutes. The tops should have set yet still be jiggly.

7. Allow it to cool. Drizzle maple syrup on top.

Nutrition Facts:

Calories: 530

Protein: 19 grams

Fat: 45 grams

Carbs: 9 grams

Pumpkin Spice Creme Brulee (Serves 2)

Ingredients:

2 Egg Yolks

1 teaspoon of Pumpkin Pie Spice

2 tablespoons of Erythritol

1 cup of Heavy Cream

2 tablespoons of Pumpkin Puree

Directions:

1. Preheat your oven to 300 degrees. Heat heavy cream in saucepan. Don't allow to boil. Add in pumpkin pie spice once your cream begins to bubble. Turn off the heat and cover with your lid. Allow to stand for 5 minutes.

2. Separate two egg yolks and then whisk until they're both light yellow.

3. Slowly add your cream mixture to your eggs while continuously whisking.

4. Once combined, add your pumpkin puree. Whisk together well.

5. Add your erythritol. Mix well.

6. Place 2 ramekins in your deep baking dish and fill with hot water (approximately 1/2 way up ramekins).

7. Pour your mixture into ramekins and bake approximately 30 to 40 minutes. Tops of creme brulees will be set but jiggly.

8. Allow it to cool for approximately 15 minutes. Place in refrigerator at least 4 hours.

9. Sprinkle erythritol on top if you desire extra sweetness.

10. Use a blowtorch to burn tops of your creme brulees. Can also place in broiler for 1 to 2 minutes if you don't have a torch.

<u>Nutrition Facts:</u>

Calories: 460

Protein: 5 grams

Fat: 49 grams

Carbs: 5 grams

Pumpkin-Spiced Chocolate Slab (Serves 12)

__Ingredients:__

4 Pumpkin Spiced Collagen Bars (Chopped Into Squares)

1 cup of Cacao Butter

1 teaspoon of Vanilla Powder

2 tablespoons of Grass-Fed Ghee

1 cup of Raw Unsweetened Cocoa Powder

Pinch of Salt

Sweetener of Choice

__Directions:__

1. Add your ghee and cacao butter to your small-sized saucepan and heat on low until completely melted.

2. Add your chocolate powder, vanilla, salt, and sweetener to taste and stir through to combine.

3. Line your small-medium sized container with baking paper.

4. Pour your liquid chocolate into the lined container. Sprinkle the chopped bars over the top of your chocolate.

5. Place in the refrigerator to set.

6. When it's ready, slice your chocolate slab into 12 even squares.

Nutrition Facts:

Calories: 234

Carbs: 15 grams

Fat: 20 grams

Quest Cookies (Serves 1)

Ingredients:

1 Quest Bar

Directions:

1. Preheat your oven to 450 degrees.

2. Microwave bar for 10 seconds.

3. Break into 8 evenly sized parts and roll up into balls.

4. Put on your baking sheet and cook for approximately 3 minutes.

Nutrition Facts:

Calories: 190

Protein: 21 grams

Fat: 8 grams

Carbs: 20 grams

Raspberry Cream Crepes

<u>Ingredients:</u>

<u>Crepes:</u>

2 Eggs

2 tablespoons of Erythritol

2 ounces of Cream Cheese

Pinch of Salt

Dash of Cinnamon

<u>Filling:</u>

1/2 cup + 2 tablespoons of Whole Milk Ricotta

3 ounces of Raspberries

<u>Toppings:</u>

Whipped Cream

Sugar-Free Maple Syrup

Directions:

1. Combine all of your crepe ingredients into your food processor or blender. Blend together for approximately 20 seconds so no chunks remain.

2. Heat your pan over medium heat. Spray with your cooking spray and put a 1/4 of your batter at a time. While pouring, tilt pan onto all sides so your crepe batter reaches each edge of the pan.

3. Let your crepe cook for approximately 1 minute. Then wedge your spatula underneath and wiggle gently until you reach the center and flip it. Let cook another 15 seconds.

4. Continue doing this process until all your batter is gone. Should make 5 or 6 crepes in total.

5. Let crepes cool. Lay next to one another not on top of each other.

6. Stuff them with your whole ricotta cheese.

7. Add your raspberries.

8. Fold each side of crepe over your filling and press down gently to seal it.

9. Add toppings.

<u>Nutrition Facts:</u>

Calories: 570

Protein: 15 grams

Fat: 40 grams

Carbs: 8 grams

Raspberry Lime Cheesecake Fat Bombs (Serves 16)

Ingredients:

1/4 cup of Melted Coconut Oil

8 drops of Liquid Stevia

4 ounces of Cream Cheese

4 tablespoons of Unsalted Butter

1/4 cup of Fresh Raspberries

Zest of 1 Lime

Juice of 1/2 a Lime

Directions:

1. In your microwave safe bowl, combine your butter and cream cheese, and microwave in 30-second intervals until your mixture is smooth and creamy but not totally melted.

2. Whisk your mixture until well-incorporated, then pour in your coconut oil and whisk vigorously.

3. Add your stevia, lime juice, and lime zest, and mix everything together.

4. Add your fresh raspberries, and crush them lightly as you whisk them in.

5. Grab a silicone mold or a mini-muffin tin with liners, and divide the mixture evenly.

6. Place in your freezer until frozen solid. Remove from the mold. Store in the freezer or they will melt.

Red Velvet Cinnamon Cheesecakes (Serves 4)

Ingredients:

Red Velvet Layer:

1 Egg

1 teaspoon of Red Food Coloring

1/4 cup of Butter

1 tablespoon of Cocoa Powder

1/2 teaspoon of Vanilla Extract

6 tablespoons of Almond Flour

1/2 teaspoon of Apple Cider Vinegar

Pinch of Salt

Cheesecake Layer:

1 Egg

1 tablespoon of Butter

2 tablespoons of Erythritol

1/2 teaspoon of Vanilla Extract

6 ounces of Cream Cheese

1 teaspoon of Cinnamon

Pinch of Salt

Directions:

Red Velvet Layer:

1. Preheat your oven to 350 degrees.

2. Melt butter in your small saucepan. Combine it with the erythritol. Keep the flame on low heat until your erythritol is dissolved.

3. In your mixing bowl, combine butter and erythritol with salt, vanilla, and cocoa powder.

4. Add in your egg and mix together until it is well combined.

5. Add in food coloring and your apple cider vinegar.

6. Add sifted almond flour and mix it together until fully combined.

7. Evenly pour your mixture among 4 greased ramekins. Be sure to tap a hard surface to flatten your batter out and remove the air bubbles. Place them on your cookie sheet and place them into your refrigerator while you're making your cheesecake layer.

Cheesecake Layer:

1. Using your electric hand mixer, beat your softened cream cheese and butter until light and fluffy.

2. Add in vanilla extract, cinnamon, and egg. Beat your mixture again.

3. Add your powdered erythritol and salt. Mix with your electric hand mixer.

Combining:

1. Take your ramekins out of refrigerator and spoon about 2 big teaspoons onto each of the red velvet layers. They shouldn't mix, but should meet without having any gaps between each of them.

2. Use your spoon to push the cheesecake layer to edges of your ramekins. Make sure there are no gaps between your ramekins and your cakes. Tap your ramekins again on a hard surface so your top layer will flatten out.

3. Bake in your oven for approximately 20 minutes. Make sure tops are set before removing from oven.

4. Allow it to cool.

Nutrition Facts:

Calories: 420

Protein: 17 grams

Fat: 36 grams

Carbs: 2 grams

Saffron Panna Cotta (Serves 6)

Ingredients:

1/2 tablespoon of Unflavored Powdered Gelatin

1/4 teaspoon of Vanilla Extract

2 cups of Heavy Whipping Cream

Pinch of Saffron

Water

1 tablespoon of Chopped Almonds (Optional)

1 tablespoon of Honey (Optional)

12 Fresh Raspberries (Optional)

Directions:

1. Mix your gelatin with a small amount of water (follow instructions for your chosen brand, usually 1 tablespoon water for every 1 teaspoon of gelatin) and set aside to bloom.

2. Bring your cream, vanilla, saffron, and optional honey to a light boil in your saucepan. Lower the heat and allow to simmer for a few minutes.

3. Remove your pan from the stove top and add your gelatin. Stir until completely dissolved.

4. Pour your mix into 6 glasses or ramekins. Cover with plastic wrap and place in your refrigerator for at least 2 hours. Toast the almonds in a dry, hot frying pan for a few minutes and add on top of the panna cotta with raspberries.

Nutrition Facts:

Calories: 271

Net Carbs: 2 grams

Salted Caramel Panna Cotta (Serves 4)

<u>Ingredients:</u>

1/4 cup of Erythritol

1/2 cup of Caramel

2 cups of Heavy Cream

1 sachet of Unflavored Gelatin

1 teaspoon of Vanilla

<u>Directions:</u>

1. Heat up your cream in a saucepan over a low heat. Add in your erythritol and gelatin. Don't allow to boil or simmer.

2. Use your whisk to stir together well. Add your vanilla extract and stir well.

3. Grease your ramekins and wipe excess with a paper towel.

4. Pour your mixture into ramekins and chill for at least 2 hours.

5. Pour 2 tablespoons of caramel over each ramekin of panna cotta.

Nutrition Facts:

Calories: 450

Protein: 2 grams

Carbs: 6 grams

Salted Toffee Nut Cups (Serves 5)

Ingredients:

5 ounces of Low-Carb Milk Chocolate

3 tablespoons of Cold Butter

3 tablespoons + 2 teaspoons of Erythritol

1/2 ounce of Chopped Raw Walnuts

Sea Salt

Directions:

1. Melt your chocolate slowly by microwaving on low power in 45 second intervals, stirring frequently, until your chocolate is melted.

2. Place 5 paper cupcake liners into your cupcake pan. Drop a dollop of chocolate into each liner and spread to evenly cover the bottom. Brush chocolate up the edges slightly with a spoon or pastry brush. Place in the freezer to harden.

3. In your microwave safe glass bowl, heat your cold butter and erythritol on low power for three minutes. You must stir the mix every 20 to 30 seconds to prevent burning! The mixture will still look very watery and will be extremely hot! Add 2 teaspoons of erythritol and stir to thicken. Add your chopped walnuts.

4. Remove your chocolate cups from the freezer and reheat the chocolate if necessary. Fill each cup with a half spoon full of toffee mixture. If the mixture begins to separate and harden, that is normal! Just stir it gently and work quickly.

5. Top each cup with your remaining chocolate and cool in the refrigerator for 1 hour.

6. Remove from cups and sprinkle with sea salt

<u>Nutrition Facts:</u>

Calories: 195

Net Carbs: 2.25 grams

Protein: 2.5 grams

Snickers & Mars Bars Fat Bombs

Ingredients:

Bottom Layer:

1 1/4 cups of Milk Chocolate Chips

1/4 cup of Peanut Butter

Nougat Layer:

1/4 cup of Unsalted Butter

1 1/2 cups of Marshmallow Fluff

1/4 cup of Evaporated Milk

1/4 cup of Peanut Butter

1 cup of Granulated Sugar

1 teaspoon of Vanilla Extract

1 1/2 cup of Chopped Salted Peanuts

Caramel Layer:

1 14-ounce bag of Caramels

1/4 cup of Whipping Cream

Top Layer:

1 1/4 cups of Milk Chocolate Chips

1/4 cup of Peanut Butter

Directions:

Bottom Layer:

1. Buy a 9x13 disposable pan and spray it with your non-stick cooking spray.

2. In a microwave-safe dish melt together your bottom layer ingredients over 90 seconds, stopping every 30 seconds to stir, or until completely melted and well combined.

3. Spread out melted peanut butter chocolate mix into your prepped disposable container, set in your refrigerator to solidify.

Nougat Layer:

1. Melt your butter in your pan over a medium heat, then add your sugar and milk and bring it to a boil. Stir well so everything dissolves nicely.

2. Cook for approximately 5 minutes, still stirring from time to time.

3. Add your fluff, peanut butter, and vanilla - keep stirring. Make it smooth.

4. Turn off your heat and fold in your peanuts (for Snickers), or don't (for Mars bar).

5. Pour and spread over your cooled and set bottom chocolate layer. Stick it back in the refrigerator for another hour.

Caramel Layer:

1. Combine your caramels and cream in your saucepan over a low heat. Stir until smooth approximately 10 minutes.

2. Pour over your nougat and return to your refrigerator for another hour.

<u>Top Layer:</u>

1. In your microwave-safe dish melt together your top layer ingredients over 90 seconds, stopping every 30 seconds to stir, or until completely melted and combined.

2. Spread melted peanut butter chocolate mix on top of other three set layers. Place back in your refrigerator to solidify one final time.

3. Carefully remove from your pan with a spatula.

4. Cut into even size bars and refrigerate.

Strawberry Pistachio Creamsicle (Serves 4)

<u>Ingredients:</u>

8 ounces of Strawberries

1/2 cup of Heavy Cream

2 ounces of Salted Pistachios

1/2 cup of Almond Milk

2 doonk scoops of Stevia

<u>Directions:</u>

1. Place popsicle molds in the freezer beforehand to accelerate freezing process.

2. Blend your heavy cream, strawberries, almond milk, and Stevia until it is fully combined. Blend for a minute.

3. Throw in pistachios and stir. Do not blend.

4. Pour your creamsicle mix into the cold popsicle molds and insert your bases. Freeze approximately 2 hours until it has set.

5. Remove your creamsicles by running hot water on the outside of molds. Gently pull out.

Nutrition Facts:

Calories: 158

Protein: 4 grams

Fat: 13 grams

Carb: 5 grams

Strawberry Rhubarb Swirl Ice Cream (Serves 6)

Ingredients:

Strawberry Rhubarb Sauce:

1/2 teaspoon of Xanthan Gum

2 tablespoons of Granulated Stevia/Erythritol Blend

1 tablespoon of Water

1 teaspoon of Lemon Juice

1/2 cup of Diced Rhubarb

1/2 cup of Sliced Strawberries

Ice Cream:

16 ounces of Heavy Whipping Cream

1/2 cup of Granulated Stevia/Erythritol Blend

1/2 tablespoon of Vanilla Extract

3/4 cup of Unsweetened Almond Milk

Directions:

Strawberry Rhubarb Sauce:

1. In your medium-sized saucepan, combine your sweetener and xanthan gum.

2. Gradually whisk in water and lemon juice until combined.

3. Add your strawberries and rhubarb and bring saucepan to a medium heat, stirring frequently.

4. Heat your mixture until the rhubarb softens (approximately 4 to 6 minutes) and then remove from the heat. Allow the sauce to cool to room temperature before adding to the ice cream.

Ice Cream:

5. In your large-sized bowl, combine your heavy whipping cream, vanilla, and sweetener.

6. Using an electric mixer, whip your mixture until stiff peaks form.

7. Gradually add your almond milk, blending between each addition. Beat mixture until it re-thickens slightly.

8. Transfer your mixture to ice cream machine and freeze per manufacturer's instructions.

9. Once your mixture has reached the creamy texture of ice cream, transfer it to a freezer-safe container. Add the strawberry rhubarb sauce and swirl together with a spoon. Cool in freezer for approximately 2 to 3 hours before serving, stirring in 30-minute increments.

<u>Nutrition Facts:</u>

Calories: 285

Net Carbs: 3.6 grams

Fat: 29 grams

Strawberry Swirl Ice Cream (Serves 6)

<u>Ingredients:</u>

3 Large Egg Yolks

1 cup of Pureed Strawberries

1 cup of Heavy Cream

1/2 teaspoon of Vanilla Extract

1/3 cup of Erythritol

1 tablespoon of Vodka (Optional)

1/8 teaspoon of Xanthan Gum (Optional)

<u>Directions:</u>

1. Set a pot with your heavy cream over a low flame to heat up. Add in your erythritol.

2. Don't let your cream boil, just let it gently simmer till the erythritol is all dissolved.

3. Separate your egg yolks into a large mixing bowl. Beat with your electric mixer until doubled in size.

4. Temper your eggs so they don't scramble, add a couple tablespoons of the heated cream mixture at a time to the eggs while you're beating them.

5. Continue until your egg mixture is warm and then add in the rest of your cream mixture slowly, beating them constantly.

6. Add your vanilla extract and mix.

7. Optional step. Add your vodka and xanthan gum.

8. Place bowl in freezer and leave for 2 hours occasionally taking out to stir, Can also churn using your ice cream maker if you have one.

9. Puree your strawberries.

10. Once the ice cream has been chilled and is beginning to thicken add in your pureed strawberries.

11. Mix in your strawberries but don't mix too much. You want ribbons of your strawberry visible in the ice cream.

12. Place in freezer for 4 to 6 hours.

Nutrition Facts:

Calories: 178

Protein: 2 grams

Fat: 17 grams

Carbs: 3 grams

Sugar-Free Lemon Curd

Ingredients:

2 Large Eggs

1/2 cup of Meyer Lemon Juice

2 Large Egg Yolks

2 tablespoons + 2 teaspoons of Truvia

6 tablespoons of Butter (Cut Into Cubes)

Directions:

1. Whisk your lemon juice, sweetener, eggs, and egg yolks together in your saucepan.

2. Add your butter and turn the heat up to a low temperature stirring continuously.

3. Once all of your butter has melted, turn the heat up to a medium-high.

4. Continue to stir until it thickens up.

5. Remove from the heat and pour through a mesh strainer to remove any egg bits.

6. Store in your refrigerator.

Sugar-Free Maple Nut Fudge (Serves 24)

Ingredients:

8-ounce package of Mascarpone or Cream Cheese

1 teaspoon of Maple Extract

1 teaspoon of Stevia Glycerite

1 cup of Organic Butter

1/4 cup of Swerve

Options:

1 cup of Pecans or Walnuts

1/4 teaspoon of Ground Ginger

Directions:

1. In your small-sized saucepan, melt butter over a medium-high heat (heat until it turns brown, not black).

2. Add natural sweeteners until sweeteners dissolve and the mixture bubbles just a little.

3. Using a hand mixer on a low speed, add in extract and mascarpone.

4. Mix until well combined.

5. The mixture will not emulsify until it cools a little. I placed the mixture into my blender and combined until smooth which caused it to not separate. If you use a hand mixer, it keeps separating until cooled. So after it cools a bit, whip it together.

6. Stir in the nuts and ginger if using.

7. Place a piece of parchment in an 8x8 square baking pan. Pour your mixture into the pan lined with parchment. Refrigerate overnight, the mixture will thicken a lot. Remove from your pan, peel away parchment and cut into 1-inch cubes. Makes 24 servings.

<u>Nutrition Facts:</u>

Carbs: 19 grams

Calories: 110

Sugar-Free Mounds Bars (Serves 24)

<u>Ingredients:</u>

1/3 cup of Organic Extra Virgin Coconut Oil

1/2 cup of Confectioner's Style Swerve

8 ounces of Dark Chocolate (85% Cacao)

1 cup of Unsweetened Organic Finely Shredded Coconut

1/3 cup of Organic Coconut Milk

<u>Directions:</u>

1. In your medium-sized saucepan, combine your coconut oil, coconut milk, and the sweetener.

2. Heat over a low heat, constantly mixing until the coconut oil has melted.

3. Add your shredded coconut and mix until well mixed.

4. Pour your mixture in a 9x5 inch silicone loaf pan. Press your mixture tightly and evenly to the bottom of your pan.

5. Refrigerate for 3 hours or until your mixture is solid.

6. Turn your pan upside down, gently press the bottom of your pan so that the solid mixture pops out.

7. Cut your mixture into bars.

8. Chop your chocolate into small-sized pieces, equal in size.

9. Melt 3 ounces of your chopped chocolate in a water bath or in a double boiler. Don't let the chocolate get too hot, heat it gently until it is melted, stirring occasionally.

10. Remove your melted chocolate from the heat. Add 1 ounce of chopped chocolate to your melted chocolate and mix occasionally to get a smooth mixture.

11. Dip your bars in the melted chocolate, put on parchment paper or on cooling rack and let the chocolate set.

12. When your chocolate coating is completely set, melt 3 ounces of the chopped chocolate in a water bath or in a double boiler. Don't let your chocolate get too hot, heat it gently until it is melted, stirring occasionally.

13. Remove the chocolate from your heat. Add the rest of your chopped chocolate (1 ounce) to your melted chocolate and mix occasionally to get a smooth mixture.

14. Dip your bars a second time in your melted chocolate, put on parchment paper or on cooling rack and allow your chocolate to set.

Nutrition Facts:

Net Carbs: 2.1 grams

Calories: 110

Sugar-Free Panna Cotta (Serves 4)

<u>Ingredients:</u>

1 cup of Unsweetened Almond Milk

1 teaspoon of Vanilla Extract

1 cup of Heavy Cream

1/2 cup of Sugar-Free Raspberry Jam

1 sachet of Unflavored Gelatin

1/3 cup of Erythritol

1 tablespoon of Fresh Lemon Juice

Raspberries

<u>Directions:</u>

1. In your saucepan, combine the almond milk and heavy cream over a low flame.

2. Add your gelatin and erythritol. Allow to dissolve in your warm cream. Don't allow to boil.

3. Use your whisk to stir it together well.

4. Turn off heat and add your lemon juice and vanilla extract.

5. Grease 4 cups or ramekins. Spray with oil and pour your batter into each one evenly.

6. Cover your cup or ramekin with plastic wrap and place in refrigerator for a minimum of 2 hours.

7. Take out and run a knife around edges. Flip over onto a plate.

8. Top with your raspberry jam and fresh raspberries.

Nutrition Facts:

Calories: 131

Fat: 12 grams

Carbs: 11 grams

Vanilla Fat Bombs (Serves 14)

Ingredients:

1 cup of Unsalted Macadamia Nuts

1 Vanilla Bean or 2 teaspoon of Sugar-Free Vanilla Extract

1/4 cup of Virgin Coconut Oil

1/4 cup of Butter

Optional:

10 to 15 drops of Stevia Extract

2 tablespoons of Swerve

Directions:

1. Place your macadamia nuts into your blender and pulse until smooth.

2. Mix with your softened butter and coconut oil (room temperature or melted in a water bath).

3. Add your swerve, stevia, and vanilla bean.

4. Pour into your mini muffin forms or an ice cube tray. You should be able to fill each one about 1 1/2 tablespoons of your mixture to get 14 servings. Place in the refrigerator for approximately 30 minutes and let it solidify.

5. When done, keep refrigerated. Coconut oil and butter get soft at room temperature.

Nutrition Facts:

Net Carbs: 0.6 grams

Calories: 132

White Chocolate Butter Pecan Bombs (Serves 4)

Ingredients:

2 tablespoons of Coconut Oil

1/4 teaspoon of Vanilla Extract

2 tablespoons of Powdered Erythritol

2 tablespoons of Butter

1/2 cup of Chopped Pecans

2 ounces of Cocoa Butter

Pinch of Stevia

Pinch of Salt

Directions:

1. Melt your coconut oil, cocoa butter, and butter together in a small-sized pan until melted. Then turn your heat off.

2. Stir in 2 tablespoons of powdered erythritol into your butter mixture until well combined.

3. Add a pinch of salt to bring out the sweetness.

4. Add a pinch of Stevia.

5. Add your vanilla extract.

6. Add a few chopped pecans into your silicone molds. Add around 3 to 4 pecans total to each mold. If you don't have pecans, walnuts and hazelnuts work well.

7. Pour your white chocolate mix evenly into the molds over your nuts and place in your freezer immediately.

8. Freeze for approximately 30 minutes.

Nutrition Facts:

Calories: 287

Carbs: 0.5 grams

Fat: 30 grams

White Chocolate Raspberry Cheesecake Fluff

Ingredients:

2 ounces of Heavy Cream

1 teaspoon of Stevia Glycerite

8 ounces of Softened Cream Cheese

1 teaspoon of Low Sugar Raspberry Preserves

1 tablespoon of Da Vinci Sugar-Free White Chocolate Flavor Syrup

Directions:

1. Mix all your ingredients together and then whip it into a pudding-like consistency. Spoon mixture into small-sized serving cups and then refrigerate until it sets.

Zabaglione w/ Meringues (Serves 6)

Ingredients:

6 Medium Organic Eggs (Yolks Divided From Whites)

3 Medium Organic Strawberries

1 stick of Organic Butter

4 tablespoons of Coconut Oil

1 gram of Powdered Stevia

2 teaspoons of Vanilla Extract (Divided)

1 cup of Heavy Whipping Cream

Zest of 1 Organic Lemon (Peeled w/ Potato Peeler)

Directions:

Meringues:

1. Pre-heat your oven to 200 degrees.

2. In your large-sized bowl place your egg whites, 1/2 of the stevia, and 1 teaspoon of vanilla extract.

3. With your hand mixer whip your egg whites, starting with a slow setting for about 30 seconds, until they become foamy, then on the fastest setting, until they get stiff and hold a peak.

4. Set to the side about 1/3 of your egg whites for later.

5. Line your cookie sheet with parchment paper.

6. Gently spoon your egg whites into a pastry bag with a large nozzle.

7. Squeeze little round mounds of egg white on your cookie sheet in a decorative fashion.

8. Set your cookie sheet in the oven and bake for approximately 3 hours with the door slightly ajar.

9. Meringues will be ready when they sound hollow when tapped.

Zabaglione:

1. Start melting your butter and coconut oil in a small-sized heat-resistant bowl, set in a small-sized saucepan of boiling water.

2. In your blender put your washed and trimmed strawberries, the zest of the lemon, the rest of your stevia and the vanilla extract.

3. Mix your eggs well, until smooth and foamy.

4. Add your strawberry mixture to them.

5. Once your butter has melted, slowly pour your egg yolk mix into your bowl, while mixing all the time with your hand mixer on the slowest setting.

6. Add the rest of your whipped egg whites in and mix gently.

7. Keep mixing the zabaglione, while holding the bowl, so it will not spin.

8. Cook for approximately 5 minutes, making sure that it does not stick to the sides of the bowl.

9. It should be light and frothy when done. Remove the bowl from the boiling water and set to the side.

Whipped Cream:

1. In a previously chilled bowl, pour your heavy cream.

2. Whip with your hand mixer on a high speed until stiff.

3. In a glass, layer the zabaglione with the meringue and top with whipped cream.

4. Serve immediately or pre-make and chill in the refrigerator.

<u>**Nutrition Facts:**</u>

Calories: 367

Fat: 36